AF818171

Annales Nestlé

Intractable Diarrheas in Childhood

Nestlé Nutrition

KARGER Basel · Freiburg · Paris · London · New York · Bangalore · Bangkok · Singapore · Tokyo · Sydney

S. Karger
Medical and Scientific Publishers
Basel • Freiburg • Paris • London
New York • Bangalore • Bangkok
Singapore • Tokyo • Sydney

Disclaimer
Nestlé Nutrition-Nestec Ltd./S. Karger AG cannot be held responsible for errors or omissions, or for any consequences arising from the use of the information contained herein.

Drug Dosage
The authors and the publisher have exerted every effort to ensure that drug selection and dosage set forth in this text are in accord with current recommendations and practice at the time of publication. However, in view of ongoing research, changes in government regulations, and the constant flow of information relating to drug therapy and drug reactions, the reader is urged to check the package insert for each drug for any change in indications and dosage and for added warnings and precautions. This is particularly important when the recommended agent is a new and/or infrequently employed drug.

Printed in Switzerland on acid-free paper by Reinhardt Druck, Basel
ISBN 3–8055–8016–9

KARGER

Fax +41 61 306 12 34
E-Mail karger@karger.ch
www.karger.com

Annales Nestlé

Vol. 64, No. 1, 2006

Contents

KARGER

Fax +41 61 306 12 34
E-Mail karger@karger.ch
www.karger.com

Access to full text and tables of contents,
including tentative ones for forthcoming issues:
www.karger.com/ane_issues

Policy Statement

The Nestlé Nutrition Institute was created to provide health professionals with up to date information on nutrition and nutrition-related disorders in order to enable them to continuously improve patient care based on the latest medical and scientific breakthroughs.

One of the key pillars of the Nestlé Nutrition Institute is the *Annales Nestlé*, a pediatric journal that has been published on a regular basis since 1942. It contains review articles on clinical practice and research in all fields of pediatrics with focus on nutrition. Each publication deals with one specific topic, such as diabetes mellitus, celiac disease, or trace element needs of infants and children. The *Annales Nestlé* comprises 3 issues each year in 5 languages (English, French, Spanish, German and Chinese), and with around 70,000 copies per issue is one of the most widely read pediatric journals in the world.

The *Annales Nestlé* is edited by an independent editorial board of four highly respected professors of pediatrics, thus guaranteeing the medical and scientific impartiality of the journal, and hence the high level of respect and appreciation in medical and scientific circles. The editorial board sets editorial policy, identifies topics to be addressed, selects authors and assesses the articles' contents.

From 2006 onwards, the *Annales Nestlé* will be published by S. Karger AG, one of the world's most highly respected scientific and medical publishers. It is our expectation that this new partnership will further enhance the impact and appreciation that the journal has enjoyed for over 60 years.

KARGER

Fax +41 61 306 12 34
E-Mail karger@karger.ch
www.karger.com

Access to full text and tables of contents, including tentative ones for forthcoming issues:
www.karger.com/ane_issues

Annales Nestlé

Ann Nestlé 2006;64:5–6
DOI: 10.1159/000087321

Editorial

'Intractable diarrheas' in infancy emerged from the medical literature 40 years ago, in the early 1960s; the term was coined to define a group of infants (less than 3 months of age) who had diarrhea for more than 14 days, had negative stool culture and whose diarrhea persisted despite medical intervention. During the following years it became apparent that this clinical entity was heterogeneous including both cases of severe post enteritis diarrhea more or less complicated by food allergy ('protracted diarrhea') and cases of diarrhea that persisted despite bowel rest during weeks or months and resisted any pharmacological treatment (steroids, loperamide, somatostatin, ...).

In developed countries, the increasing hygiene standards and the liberal use of formulas made of partially hydrolyzed (peptides, oligosaccharides) or easily absorbable (MCT) nutrients by mouth or via constant rate enteral nutrition allowed the first subgroup of patients to eventually be cured. On the contrary, the development of total parenteral nutrition favored the emergence of a small residual group of patients who would have died before the advent of this intensive care technique.

Indeed, it is from the late 1970s, early 1980s that the various entities that will be discussed in this issue of the *Annales Nestlé* were described for the first time. Ten years later a careful analysis of these patients using both clinical and immunohistochemical criteria enabled the design of algorithms that would help to differentiate enteropathies due to congenital enterocyte defects, the earliest and most severe ones from those secondary to an abnormal (sometimes congenital) immune activation of lamina propria T cells and occurring usually somewhat later (usually before the end of the second year) in the life of the child.

The long-term treatment of these children is one of the greatest challenges facing pediatric gastroenterology: although home total parenteral nutrition allows some of these children to live a nearly normal life, it is often complicated by episodes of life-threatening central catheter-linked sepsis, the progressive shortage of venous access, and above all hepatic failure. These risks, which were recognized as TPN developed, led early to the project of small bowel transplantation which, however, has only recently come to maturity. It is now a reasonable alternative to TPN in these cases of intestinal failure.

It is the fascinating history of this recent chapter of pediatric gastroenterology that this issue of *Annales Nestlé* wishes to bring to its readers.

Alan D. Phillips from the Centre for Paediatric Gastroenterology of the Royal Free Hospital, in London, UK, is one of those who first described the anatomical (histological and ultrastructural) lesions of the congenital enterocyte defects responsible for the most severe forms of intractable diarrhea, and particularly of familial microvillous atrophy (or microvillous inclusion disease). The later condition summarizes the problems raised by these diarrheas: extreme severity (up to 300 ml/kg/day of stool output), difficulties in maintaining water and electrolyte balance and a normal growth while preventing hepatic failure, inescapable discussion of intestinal transplantation.

KARGER

Fax +41 61 306 12 34
E-Mail karger@karger.ch
www.karger.com

0517–8606/06/0641–0005$23.50/0

Accessible online at:
www.karger.com/ane

Philip M. Sherman and Ernest Cutz from the Hospital for Sick Children in Toronto, Canada, and Olivier Goulet from Necker-Enfants Malades Hospital in Paris, France, present the main features of the other group of intractable diarrhea due to immune or autoimmune enteropathies. The great interest of differentiating this group of patients from the previous one is that, although it may also induce extremely severe diarrhea (usually in somewhat older children), the therapeutic approach, once the diagnosed is made, is completely different, based on the use of immunosuppressive drugs and, in the most severe cases (IPEX syndrome), on bone marrow transplantation.

Olivier Goulet from Necker-Enfants Malades Hospital in Paris, France, participated in the description of some of these new entities (epithelial dysplasia, syndromatic diarrhea) and is a leader in the field of intestinal transplantation. He introduces the concept of intestinal failure, the ultimate consequence of these intractable diarrheas, as well as other anatomical situations (short bowel syndrome in particular), which often would impose intestinal transplantation. However, he shows here that whereas intestinal transplantation did not raise unusual technical difficulties, it did raise serious immunological problems until the advent of immunosuppressor drugs such as tacrolimus, which recently allowed this transplantation to reach acceptable 1-year survival rates.

Finally Zulfiqar A. Bhutta from the Department of Paediatrics and Child Health of the Aga Khan University in Karachi, Pakistan, usefully recalls that, in developing countries, most cases of protracted diarrhea still occur as a complication of infectious diarrhea linked to preexisting malnutrition, micronutrient deficiency, decreased immune defenses, inadequate treatment, elevated infectious burden. He shows that protracted diarrhea is the background from which the rare cases of intractable diarrheas described in the Western world emerged. After having precisely reviewed our current knowledge concerning the mechanisms leading to protracted diarrhea, Zulfiqar A. Bhutta summarizes the rules to be followed to avoid such situations.

It is hoped that this issue of *Annales Nestlé* will help all pediatricians to prevent diarrhea from becoming protracted, and to recognize and correctly take in charge the rare cases that are intractable and need the assistance of specialized teams dedicated to their long-term treatment.

The Editorial Committee

Annales Nestlé

Ann Nestlé 2006;64:7–13
DOI: 10.1159/000086495

Immune and Autoimmune Enteropathies

Philip M. Sherman[a] Ernest Cutz[a] Olivier Goulet[b]

[a]Hospital for Sick Children, University of Toronto, Toronto, Ont., Canada; [b]Groupe Hospitalier Necker-Enfant Malade, Paris, France

Key Words

Diarrhea, children and infants · Enteropathy, immune and autoimmune · IPEX syndrome · Autoimmunity

Abstract

Autoimmune enteropathy characteristically presents in infancy with protracted diarrhea. Underlying disorders of immune function, including regulatory T cells, must be excluded. Treatment options include nutritional rehabilitation, immune suppression, and, in select cases, bone marrow transplant.

Introduction

Autoimmune enteropathy and enteropathies due to primary immune deficiencies are relatively uncommon causes of protracted diarrhea during infancy. When confronted with an infant or young child with chronic unexplained diarrhea, the differential diagnosis is quite extensive [1] and distinct from the considerations in assessing an adult with the same clinical symptoms [2, 3]. In most parts of the world, infectious and post-infectious enteropathies remain the most common causes of protracted diarrhea [4]. Some investigators contend that allergic enteropathies also are common in young children, even in the absence of other atopic symptoms or a family history of an allergic predisposition. Much more commonly, milk and soy protein-induced allergic colitis develops in newborns and infants, including those receiving breast milk as their sole source of nutrients. In an older child who has received gluten in the diet, it is important to consider celiac disease as the underlying cause of symptoms since it is increasingly apparent that gluten-sensitive enteropathy has protean manifestations and is a life-long condition that can be treated effectively and safely with appropriate dietary adjustments [5].

One helpful way to consider alternative etiologies is to differentiate those causes of chronic diarrhea in which there is a relatively intact villus-crypt unit from those with abnormal villus-crypt architecture (i.e. an enteropathy). In the former scenario, conditions such as congenital disorders of ion transport and secretory diarrhea, due to bacterial enterotoxins and hormone-secreting tumors, need to be considered [1]. By contrast, an enteropathy with a reduction in villus height should bring to mind a completely different set of diagnostic considerations. After infectious and allergic etiologies have been excluded, chronic high volume diarrhea beginning in the first few days of life should raise microvillus inclusion disease for diagnostic consideration [6]. This latter condition also is referred to as familial microvillous atrophy [7] or Davidson's syndrome.

KARGER

Fax +41 61 306 12 34
E-Mail karger@karger.ch
www.karger.com

0517–8606/06/0641–0007$23.50/0

Accessible online at:
www.karger.com/ane

Philip M. Sherman, MD, FRCPC
Gastroenterology and Nutrition, Room 8409
Hospital for Sick Children, 555 University Avenue
Toronto, Ont. M5G 1X8 (Canada)
Tel. +1 416 813 7734, Fax +1 416 813 6531, E-Mail philip.sherman@sickkids.ca

With slightly later onset of chronic diarrhea, a condition that can present much like autoimmune enteropathy is tufting enteropathy [8], which also is referred to as intestinal epithelial dysplasia [9]. Interestingly, many of the infants reported from both Europe and North America with this enteropathy are from families originally from North Africa, Turkey and, especially, the island of Malta. As a result, tufting enteropathy certainly should be considered seriously in infants of these backgrounds.

Clinical Presentation

Children with autoimmune enteropathy typically present after the neonatal period, but within the first year of life. A history of maternal polyhydramnios during the pregnancy and/or a family history of other affected children should direct a search for other causes of protracted diarrhea of neonatal onset including, for example, congenital chloride-losing enteropathy [1].

Most cases of autoimmune enteropathy begin with chronic, watery and unremitting diarrhea between 2 and 4 months of age after an uneventful pregnancy and neonatal period. However, the later onset of symptoms is well described, including isolated case reports of initial manifestations of diarrheal disease during adolescence [10] and the adult years [11]. These older-onset patients typically carry the diagnosis of refractory sprue, until an analysis for the presence of anti-enterocyte antibodies is carried out. It remains to be established whether the later onset of symptoms is due to the same molecular basis of disease as for those with the development of diarrhea during the first year of life.

Although such autoimmune conditions primarily manifest as enteropathies, the colon often is involved as well. Signs and symptoms of colitis (for example: urgency, tenesmus, hematochezia and mucus in the stools) accompanying protracted diarrhea that is unresponsive to a trial of elemental feeding – particularly in association with impaired growth and undernutrition – should raise the suspicion of an autoimmune enteropathy.

The presence of other autoimmune conditions also raises the risk of autoimmune enteropathy. Initial cases of autoimmune enteropathy described in the scientific literature were associated with type-1 diabetes mellitus, autoimmune thyroiditis, autoimmune hemolytic anemia and skin conditions that likely had an autoimmune basis. Many of the affected cases reported also were associated with tubulonephropathy.

Histopathologic Findings

Small bowel biopsies in infants and children with protracted diarrhea are extremely helpful. Results of morphology and immunohistochemistry are not only helpful in establishing a specific diagnosis, but frequently also can exclude other conditions when such evaluations are not definitive [12].

In cases of autoimmune enteropathy, light microscopy findings (fig. 1a) often resemble many of the features associated with gluten-sensitive enteropathy even when affected children have not been challenged with gluten. Examinations of sections stained with hematoxylin and eosin often reveal total villus atrophy and crypt hyperplasia. In addition, there often is marked immune cell infiltration including activated T cells [13], into the lamina propria of the intestinal mucosa. There also can be morphological evidence of intraepithelial lymphocytes, but not to the same degree as that observed in children with total villus atrophy caused by celiac disease [14]. Immunohistochemistry, with relevant antibodies as markers, provides evidence of a marked infiltration of CD3+ T cells into the lamina propria (fig. 1b). Recent findings indicate that the cytokine interleukin-21 may mediate T-cell activation, impaired survival of the cells and ultimately predispose the affected host to autoimmune diseases [15].

Colonic biopsies also show evidence of immune cells infiltrating the lamina propria in children with autoimmune enteropathy. This finding is in contrast to other causes of protracted diarrhea in infants in whom evidence of immune activation other than in the small bowel is not observed [14].

Autoantibodies

A hallmark of autoimmune enteropathy is the presence in serum of immunoglobulin G antibodies, usually circulating in low titer, which bind to apical aspect of enterocytes (fig. 2). In one report on 25 children with unexplained chronic diarrhea, anti-enterocyte antibodies were detected in 14 (56%) subjects, compared with positive test results in 3 (5%) of 53 patients with chronic inflammatory bowel diseases, 0 of 10 with celiac disease and none of the 50 children with other conditions unrelated to the gastrointestinal tract [16]. The antibody is not specific to an epitope on human enterocytes, because the autoantibodies also bind to small bowel epithelial cells in intestinal sections obtained from rats, mice and guinea pigs. The antigen also is detected in renal epithelium.

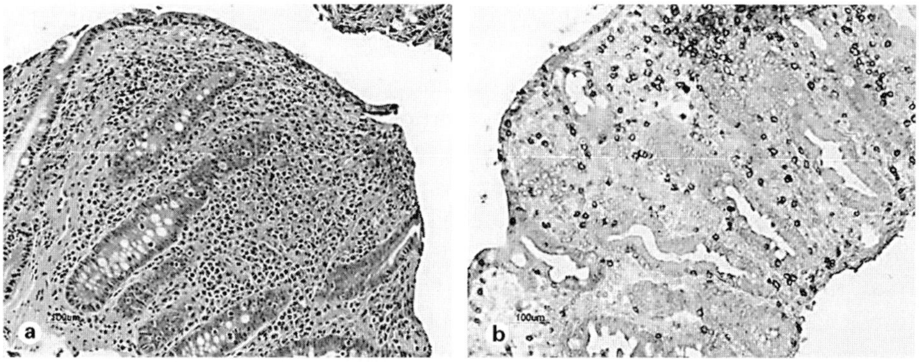

Fig. 1. a Biopsy of the small bowel mucosa obtained from a child with protracted diarrhea. The biopsy shows total villus atrophy with crypt hyperplasia and infiltration of the lamina propria by a mixed chronic inflammatory cell infiltrate. HE. Approximate original magnification ×20. **b** Immunohistochemistry with anti-CD3 antibody demonstrates infiltration of the lamina propria by numerous CD3+ T cells. Approximate original magnification ×20.

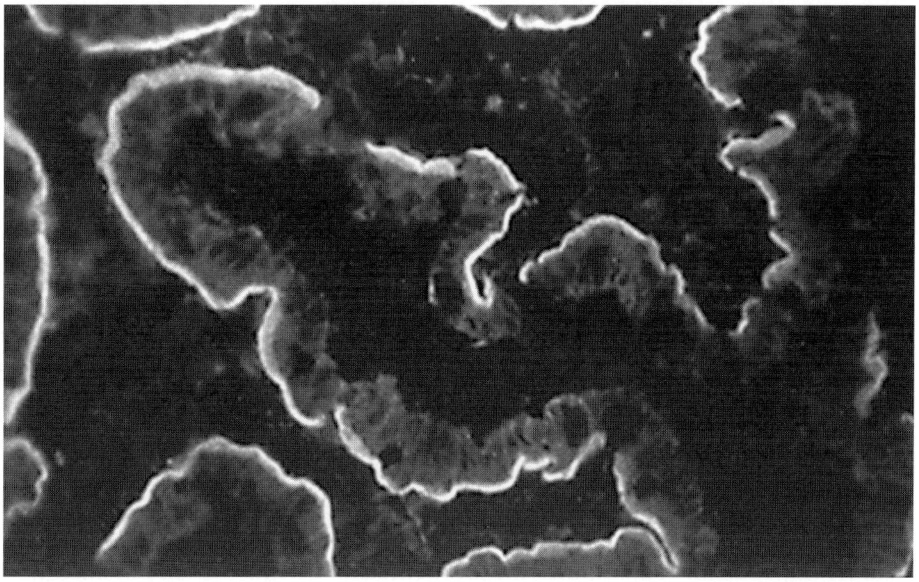

Fig. 2. Indirect immune fluorescence demonstrates the presence of anti-enterocyte antibodies in the serum of a child with autoimmune enteropathy. Fluorescent staining outlines the apical surface of enterocytes along the villus-crypt unit.

Western blots show that autoantigens are either 55 [17] or 75 kDa [18, 19]. The 75-kDa autoantigen is expressed in the small bowel, large intestine, pancreas and kidney [20]. With therapy (considered below), titers of circulating anti-enterocyte antibodies are reduced, or disappear progressively and completely with clinical improvement. Therefore, systemic autoantibody levels can be monitored as an objective measure of responsiveness to clinical interventions [17].

Even though molecular targets for anti-enterocyte antibodies have been described, other investigators observed that the test may not be sufficiently specific. For instance, Martin-Villa et al. [21] noted the presence of such autoantibodies in the systemic circulation of subjects without villous atrophy and with no history of diarrhea. Thus as with any other screening tests, these anti-enterocyte antibody assessments must be placed in appropriate clinicopathological contexts.

A few case reports describe an autoimmune enteropathy in which systemic autoantibodies are directed against the goblet cell lineage rather than apical regions of enterocytes [22]. Intestinal biopsies in these cases show a lack of goblet, Paneth and enteroendocrine cells [23]. This may reflect a deficiency in the transcription factor, Math1 [24]. The clinical and pathological findings are otherwise similar to those in other cases of autoimmune enteropathy. This finding supports the view that infiltrating T cells, rather than the systemic autoantibodies, are involved in mediating the disease's pathobiology. Thus, autoantibodies likely provide markers of an underlying condition which develops as a result of mucosal inflammation and injury, rather than being specifically involved in disease pathogenesis [13, 14].

Primary Immune Deficiency Disorders

A variety of immune disorders of genetic origin can cause intestinal injury resulting in enteropathy, malabsorption of nutrients, and protracted diarrhea [25]. For instance, chronic granulomatous disease and glycogen storage disease type 1b both have been associated with mucosal inflammation along the length of the gastrointestinal tract, with clinical, radiological, and endoscopic features that can mimic those observed in chronic inflammatory bowel diseases. Eosinophilic gastroenteritis also should be considered in the differential diagnosis.

It is now clear that there are multiple causes of what previously had been lumped together in the single entity referred to as autoimmune enteropathy. For example, primary T-cell immune deficiencies are reported to present with features of autoimmune disease. For instance, Arniaz-Villena et al. [26] reported a kindred in which there was a congenital defect in the expression of the CD3-γ subunit of the T-cell receptor complex. The affected proband presented with protracted diarrhea in association with autoantibodies against gut epithelial cells, smooth muscle and mitochondria, as well as autoimmune hemolytic anemia and a selective IgG2 subclass deficiency.

Two children with Schimke immuno-osseous dysplasia and abnormal T-cell immune function were described in the literature [27, 28]. Both children presented with chronic diarrhea and signs and symptoms consistent with autoimmune enteropathy. However, autoantibodies were not present and atypical *Mycobacteria* were identified in the small bowel mucosa in one child [28]. This observation serves to reinforce and highlight the importance of excluding chronic infection and underlying immunodeficiency state in a child with unexplained protracted diarrhea.

IPEX Syndrome

Immune dysregulation, polyendocrinopathy, enteropathy, and X-linked (IPEX) syndrome is the most specific and well-documented underlying cause of autoimmune enteropathy. The disease is caused by mutations in the *Foxp3* gene carried in the peri-centromeric region of the X chromosome: Xp11.23–Xp13.3 [29, 30]. *Foxp3* (also variously referred to as *JM2* and *scurfin*) is a transcription factor that is critical for control of the normal development of regulatory T cells [31, 32]. When mutated, the normal control of CD25+ T cells is lost [33, 34] and there is an inappropriate activation and dissemination of activated immune cells to multiple organs, including the intestinal tract (fig. 3).

Several *FoxP3* gene mutations have been reported that cause human disease. There is probably a genotype-phenotype relationship explaining differences observed in terms of clinical expression, disease severity, number of extra-digestive autoimmune manifestations, and prognoses [35]. As a result, autoimmune enteropathy can be subdivided into those cases due to IPEX, affected males without evidence of a mutation in the *FoxP3* gene, and affected girls [36].

Male infants with IPEX syndrome present in infancy with type-1 diabetes mellitus, autoimmune thyroiditis, autoimmune hemolytic anemia (positive direct Coomb's test) and a variety of skin lesions, including eczema, an ichthyosiform dermatitis, psoriatic dermatitis and alopecia universalis [37]. Protracted high-volume diarrhea, due to an autoimmune enteropathy, is generally a prominent presenting feature. These children also may present with atopic features, including food allergies, peripheral eosinophilia and raised levels of immunoglobulin E [38]. Cases of autoimmune enteropathy occurring in boys (especially if there are multiply affected siblings in the same family) with evidence of autoantibodies directed against other organs and evidence of systemic autoimmune diseases, which have been published previously in the medical literature, should be considered as possible cases of IPEX syndrome.

Therapeutic Considerations

The initial management of infants with chronic diarrhea in whom autoimmune enteropathy is a diagnostic consideration is precisely the same as that for all other affected individuals. The initial focus should target the maintenance of intravascular volume and nutritional rehabilitation, which generally requires either continuous elemental, enteral venous infusion or total parental alimentation. Children often are left dehydrated and undernourished during extensive in-hospital diagnostic evaluations. This approach is deplorable: fluid and nourishment are among the first priorities [39]. Only after these are provided should health care providers pause to consider the long list of potential considerations in the differential diagnosis.

Autoimmune enteropathy generally responds well to potent suppression of the hosts' immune system. High-dose systemic corticosteroids frequently will reduce mu-

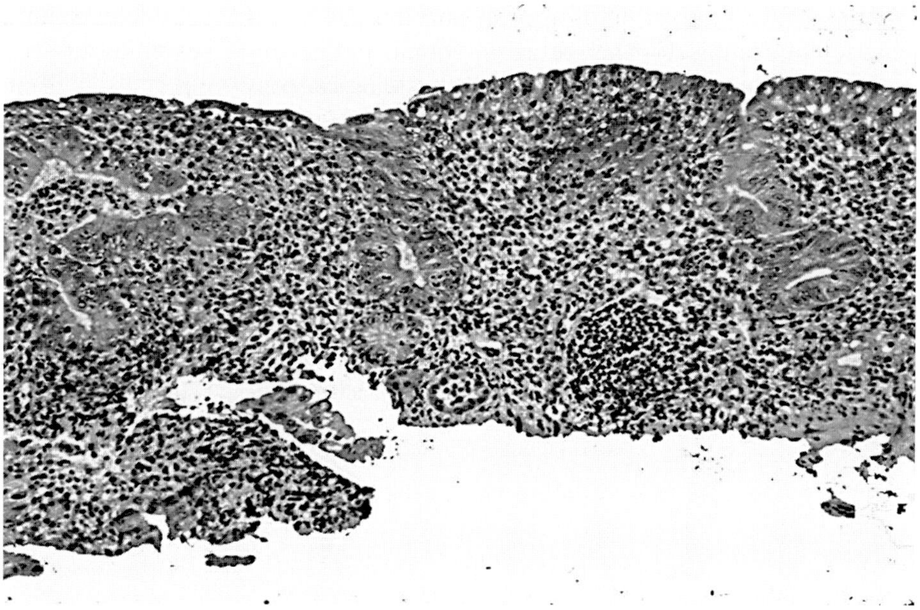

Fig. 3. Histology of the small bowel in a child with IPEX syndrome shows evidence of total villous atrophy and marked inflammation of the lamina propria with a chronic inflammatory cell infiltrate.

cosal inflammation, lower stool output and permit increased enteral delivery of calories. Autoantibody titers are reduced in parallel with clinical responses to medical therapies. However, steroid dependence (that is, recurrence of symptoms following a tapering of the corticosteroid dose) is the norm. Steroid resistance (i.e. absence of an apparent response to therapy) is also common. As a result, a number of other potent immune-suppressive agents have been employed. Case reports indicate apparent clinical benefits of a variety of therapies such as cyclosporine [40, 41], tacrolimus [42], sirolimus [43], mycophenolate mofetil [44], cyclophosphamide [45] and biologic agents such as the chimeric monoclonal antibody against tumor necrosis factor-α, infliximab [46].

Most affected children respond to potent suppression of the immune system and, ultimately, tolerate advancing enteral feedings and concurrent reductions in parenteral nutritional supports. As a result, autoimmune enteropathy should not be considered as an indication for undertaking small bowel transplant. This clinical prognosis stands in stark contrast to most cases of microvillus inclusion disease where there is no response to potent immune suppression and the outcome is guarded in the absence of intestinal transplantation, at least as a therapeutic option [1, 6, 12] .

Whether these children may benefit from alternate therapeutic strategies, such as bone marrow transplantation, is not known. Reported benefits of transplanting bone marrow-derived cells in children with IPEX syndrome [47] suggest that this approach is worth further consideration in severely affected cases with a limited or partial response to potent suppression of the immune system. Positive responses of children with IPEX syndrome to allogeneic bone marrow transplantation also emphasize the critical importance of establishing the correct underlying diagnosis of protracted diarrhea in infants and young children. Lumping affected cases together as so-called intractable diarrhea of infancy is unhelpful and may impair consideration of appropriate therapeutic options.

Careful consideration of the precise etiology of protracted diarrhea is also essential in considering genetic counseling of families with affected children. Most cases of autoimmune enteropathy appear to be sporadic without other affected family members or evidence of parental consanguinity. On the other hand, IPEX syndrome is an X-linked condition. This raises other issues related to risk in affected families that are beyond this review.

Conclusions

Autoimmune enteropathy is a term used to describe a relatively uncommon cause of protracted diarrhea in infants. This is a severe inflammatory condition, which generally is responsive to immune suppression therapy. It is quite likely that autoimmune enteropathies encompass a number of etiologies that require better definitions to enable future targeting of appropriate therapies and genetic counseling. Further research should define underlying immune disorders and pathophysiological processes that result in the disease's clinical manifestations. Appropriate relevant animal models likely will prove to be exceptionally helpful in the disease processes' delineation.

To identify genetic mutations accounting for autoimmune enteropathy, fibroblasts from a skin biopsy should be immortalized for cell culture. Similarly, messenger RNA should be isolated from intestinal biopsies for use in whole genome scanning, which is already technologically feasible and economically viable as a powerful research tool [48]. An international collaborative research effort also will improve the current understanding of the molecular basis of chronic immune-mediated enteropathies.

Acknowledgments

P.M.S. is the recipient of a Canada Research Chair in Gastrointestinal Disease. Work in the authors' laboratories is funded by operating grants from the Canadian Institutes of Health Research.

References

1 Sherman PM, Mitchell DJ, Cutz E: Neonatal enteropathies: defining the causes of protracted diarrhea of infancy. J Pediatr Gastroenterol Nutr 2004;38:16–26.
2 Camilleri M: Chronic diarrhea: a review on pathophysiology and management for the clinical gastroenterologist. Clin Gastroenterol Hepatol 2004;2:198–206.
3 Schiller LR: Chronic diarrhea. Gastroenterology 2004;127:287–293.
4 Bhutta ZA, Ghishan F, Lindley K, Memon IA, Mittal S, Rhoads JM: Persistent and chronic diarrhea and malabsorption: Working Group report of the second World Congress of Pediatric Gastroenterology, Hepatology, and Nutrition. J Pediatr Gastroenterol Nutr 2004; 39(suppl 2):S711–S716.
5 Hill ID, Dirks MH, Liptak GS, et al: Guideline for the diagnosis and treatment of celiac disease in children: recommendations of the North American Society for Pediatric Gastroenterology, Hepatology and Nutrition. J Pediatr Gastroenterol Nutr 2005;40:1–19.
6 Cutz E, Rhoads JM, Drumm B, et al: Microvillus inclusion disease: an inherited defect of brush-border assembly and differentiation. N Engl J Med 1989;320:646–651.
7 Phillips AD, Schmitz J: Familial microvillous atrophy: a clinicopathological survey of 23 cases. J Pediatr Gastroenterol Nutr 1992;14: 380–396.
8 Reifen RM, Cutz E, Griffiths AM, et al: Tufting enteropathy: a newly recognized clinicopathological entity associated with refractory diarrhea in infants. J Pediatr Gastroenterol Nutr 1994;18:379–385.
9 Patey N, Scoazec JY, Cuenod-Jabri B, et al: Distribution of cell adhesion molecules in infants with intestinal epithelial dysplasia (tufting enteropathy). Gastroenterology 1997;113: 833–843.
10 Pirisi-Hauck NC, Foss H-D, Baier J, Kurunczi S: Simultaneous occurrence of autoimmune enteropathy and recurrent deep vein thrombosis. J Pediatr Gastroenterol Nutr 2000;30:324–329.
11 Carroccio A, Volta U, Di Prima L, et al: Autoimmune enteropathy and colitis in an adult patient. Dig Dis Sci 2003;48:1600–1606.
12 Cutz E, Sherman PM, Davidson GP: Enteropathies associated with protracted diarrhea of infancy: clinicopathological features, cellular and molecular mechanisms. Pediatr Pathol Lab Med 1997;17:335–368.
13 Murch SH, Fertleman CR, Rodrigues C, et al: Autoimmune enteropathy with distinct mucosal features in T-cell activation deficiency: the contribution of T cells to the mucosal lesion. J Pediatr Gastroenterol Nutr 1999;28:393–399.
14 Cuenod B, Brousse N, Goulet O, et al: Classification of intractable diarrhea of infancy using clinical and immunohistological criteria. Gastroenterology 1990;99:1037–1043.
15 King C, Lic A, Koelsch K, Sarvetnick N: Homeostatic expansion of T cells during immune insufficiency generates autoimmunity. Cell 2004;117:265–277.
16 Mirakian R, Richardson A, Milla PJ, et al: Protracted diarrhoea of infancy: evidence in support of an autoimmune variant. Br Med J (Clin Res Ed) 1986;293:1132–1136.
17 Colletti RB, Guillot AP, Rosen S, et al: Autoimmune enteropathy and nephropathy with circulating anti-epithelial cell antibodies. J Pediatr 1991;118:858–864.
18 Kobayashi I, Imamura K, Yamada M, et al. A 75-kD autoantigen recognized by sera from patients with X-linked autoimmune enteropathy associated with nephropathy. Clin Exp Immunol 1998;111:527–531.
19 Kobayashi I, Imamura K, Kubota M, et al: Identification of an autoimmune enteropathy-related 75-kilodalton antigen. Gastroenterology 1999;117:823–830.
20 Ishikawa S, Kobayashi I, Hamada J-I, et al: Interaction of MCC2, a novel homologue of MCC tumor suppressor, with PDZ-domain protein AIE-75. Gene 2001;267:101–110.
21 Martin-Villa JM, Regueiro JR, De Juan D, et al: T-lymphocyte dysfunctions occurring together with apical gut epithelial cell autoantibodies. Gastroenterology 1991;101:390–397.
22 Moore L, Xu X, Davidson G, et al: Autoimmune enteropathy with anti-goblet cell antibodies. Hum Pathol 1995;26:1162–1168.
23 Shaoul R, Hong D, Okada Y, Cutz E, Marcon M: Lineage development in a patient without goblet, Paneth and enteroendocrine cells, a clue for intestinal epithelial differentiation. Pediatr Res 2005, in press.
24 Yang Q, Berminham A, Finegold MJ, et al: Requirement of Math1 for secretory cell lineage commitment in the mouse intestine. Science 2001;294:2155–2158.
25 Goulet O, Seidman E: Gastrointestinal manifestations of immunodeficiency. 1. Primary immunodeficiency diseases; in Walker W, Goulet O, Kleinman R, Sherman P, Shneider B, Sanderson I (eds): Pediatric Gastrointestinal Disease, ed 4. Philadelphia, B.C. Decker, 2004, pp 707–733.
26 Arniaz-Villena A, Timon M, Corell A, et al: Primary immunodeficiency caused by mutations in the gene encoding the CD3-gamma subunit of the T-lymphocyte receptor. N Engl J Med 1992;327:529–533.
27 Kaitila I, Savilahti E, Ormala T: Autoimmune enteropathy in Schimke immunoosseous dysplasia. Am J Med Genet 1998;77:427–430.
28 Stormon M, Friedman J, King S, Cutz E, Furuya KN: An unusual case of diarrhea in Schimke immuno-osseous dysplasia. J Pediatr Gastroenterol Nutr 2002;35:369–371.

29 Bennett CL, Christie J, Ramsdell F, et al: The immune dysregulation, polyendocrinopathy, enteropathy, X-linked syndrome (IPEX) is caused by mutations of FOXP3. Nat Genet 2001;27:20–21.
30 Ochs HD, Ziegler SF, Torgerson TR: FOXP3 acts as a rheostat of the immune response. Immunol Rev 2005;203:156–164.
31 Hori S, Nomura T, Sakaguchi S: Control of regulatory T cell development by the transcription factor FOXP3. Science 2003;299:1057–1061.
32 Hori S, Sakaguchi S: Foxp3: a critical regulator of the development and function of regulatory T cells. Microbes Infect 2004;6:745–751.
33 Fontenot JD, Gavin MA, Rudensky AY: FOXP3 programs the development and function of CD4+CD25+ regulatory T cells. Nat Immunol 2003;4:330–336.
34 Bakke AC, Purtzer MZ, Wildin RS: Prospective immunological profiling in a case of immune dysregulation, polyendocrinopathy, enteropathy, X-linked syndrome (IPEX). Clin Exp Immunol 2004;137:373–378.
35 Eisenbarth GS, Gottlieb PA: Autoimmune polyendocrine syndromes. N Engl J Med 2004; 350:2068–2079.
36 Ruemmele FM, Brousse N, Goulet O: Autoimmune enteropathy: molecular concepts. Curr Opin Gastroenterol 2004;20:587–591.
37 Nieves DS, Phipps RP, Pollock SJ, et al: Dermatologic and immunologic findings in the immune dysregulation, polyendocrinopathy, enteropathy, X-linked syndrome. Arch Dermatol 2004;140:466–472.
38 Patel DD: Escape from tolerance in the human X-linked autoimmunity-allergic disregulation syndrome and the Scurfy mouse. J Clin Invest 2001;107:155–157.
39 Lo CW, Walker WA: Chronic protracted diarrhea of infancy: a nutritional disease. Pediatrics 1983;72:786–800.
40 Seidman EG, Lacaille F, Russo P, et al: Successful treatment of autoimmune enteropathy with cyclosporine. J Pediatr 1990;117:929–932.
41 Sanderson IR, Phillips AD, Spencer J, Walker-Smith JA: Response to autoimmune enteropathy to cyclosporin A therapy. Gut 1991;32: 1421–1425.
42 Bousvaros A, Leichtner AM, Book L, et al: Treatment of pediatric autoimmune enteropathy with tacrolimus (FK506). Gastroenterology 1996;111:237–243.
43 Bindl L, Torgerson T, Perroni L, Youssef N, Ochs HD, Goulet O, Ruemmele FM: Successful use of the new immune-suppressor sirolimus in IPEX (immune dysregulation, polyendocrinopathy, enteropathy, X-linked syndrome). J Pediatr 2005, in press.
44 Quiroz-Tejeira RE, Ament ME, Vargas JH: Induction of remission in a child with autoimmune enteropathy using mycophenolate mofetil. J Pediatr Gastroenterol Nutr 2003;36: 482–485.
45 Oliva-Hemper MM, Loeb DM, Abraham SC, et al: Remission of severe autoimmune enteropathy after treatment with high-dose cyclophosphamide. J Pediatr Gastroenterol Nutr 2003;36:639–643.
46 Vanderhoof JA, Young RJ: Autoimmune enteropathy in a child: response to infliximab therapy. J Pediatr Gastroenterol Nutr 2002;34: 312–316.
47 Baud O, Goulet O, Canioni D, et al: Treatment of the immune dysregulation, polyendocrinopathy, enteropathy, X-linked sydrome (IPEX) by allogeneic bone marrow transplantation. N Engl J Med 2001;344:1758–1762.
48 Collins SM, McHugh K, Croitoru K, et al: The establishment of a national tissue bank for inflammatory bowel disease research in Canada. Can J Gastroenterol 2003;17:107–109.

Annales Nestlé

Ann Nestlé 2006;64:15–23
DOI: 10.1159/000086496

Intractable Diarrhoea due to Congenital Enterocyte Defects

Alan D. Phillips

Centre for Paediatric Gastroenterology, Royal Free Hospital, London, UK

Key Words
Intractable diarrhoea · Infancy · Enteropathy

Abstract
Background: Intractable diarrhoea of infancy represents a severe problem with a high degree of morbidity and mortality. These cases demand dedicated care from both parents and medical staff as there are no easy remedies. The rarity of patients indicates that progress in understanding these disorders requires concerted international efforts to pool resources and patients. Regular reviews of publications in the field are required to disseminate advances and to air hypotheses and diagnostic criteria. ***Methods:*** This is a review of current and previous literature on congenital enterocyte defects. ***Results:*** Discrete diagnoses are possible within this syndrome, and diagnostic criteria are becoming accepted. Cases are being reported on a world-wide basis, and differences in clinical course are becoming apparent with amelioration of severity in some instances. However, a high level of morbidity and mortality remains. ***Conclusions:*** There is still a long way to go in determining the underlying basis of the disorders. However, the promise of determining the genetic basis of the diseases is becoming a reality as molecular genetic analyses are performed. This is a priority as it should afford clearer diagnostic criteria, clarify disease relationships and give much need pathogenic information.

Introduction

Intractable diarrhoea remains a severe paediatric problem with a high degree of morbidity and mortality. It represents a spectacular individual burden that defies treatment. It demands committed care from both parents and medical staff. This particular course of intractable diarrhoea, i.e. congenital enterocyte defects, often affects young infants in the first days of life. Complexities that relate to tissue and venous access for diagnosis and treatment add significantly to the problems presented by diarrhoeal losses that can amount to 10% or more of body weight per day. Nevertheless, discrete diagnoses are possible. Parenteral nutrition has allowed relatively long-term survival to occur; intestinal transplantation offers hopes for a disease-free existence, and molecular genetics is being applied in an attempt to unravel the gene defects that surely lie at the basis of the disease.

KARGER
Fax +41 61 306 12 34
E-Mail karger@karger.ch
www.karger.com

0517–8606/06/0641–0015$23.50/0

Accessible online at:
www.karger.com/ane

Alan D. Phillips, PhD
Centre for Paediatric Gastroenterology
Lower 3rd Floor, Royal Free Hospital, Pond Street
London, NW3 2QG (UK)
Tel. +44 207 830 2783, Fax +44 207 830 2146, E-Mail a.phillips@medsch.ucl.ac.uk

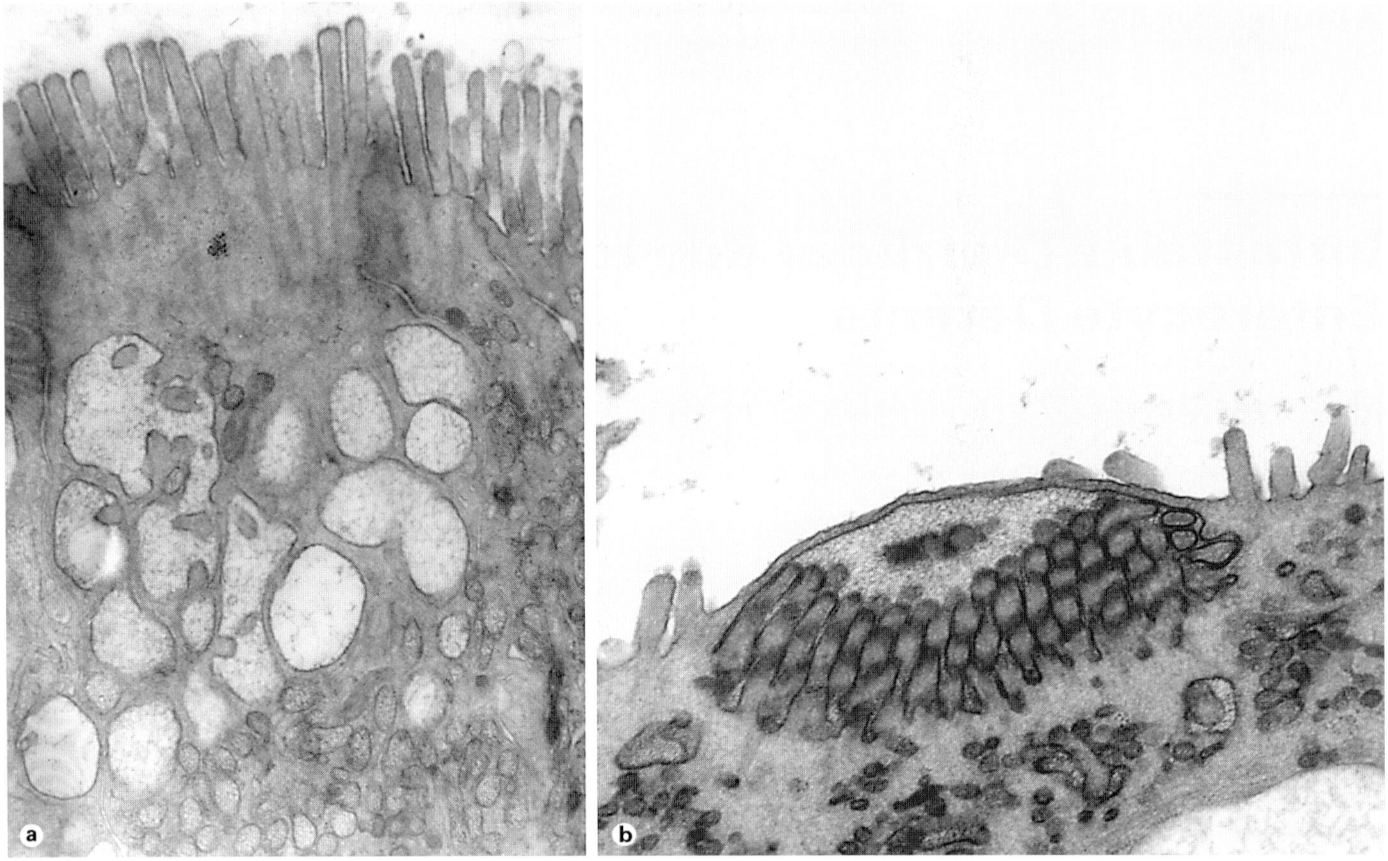

Fig. 1. Microvillous atrophy. **a** Apparent development of microvilli within a cell with an intact, although short, brush border. **b** Blister-like microvillous inclusion, appearance of engulfment.

The term intractable diarrhoea was introduced by Avery et al. [1] in the early 1960s. A group of 20 children <3 months of age with chronic diarrhoea (more than 14 days duration), negative stool cultures, and persistent diarrhoea despite medical interventions were studied. All required parenteral nutrition and 9 died. Similar reports were made in the following years [2, 3] with the suggestions that the condition was inherited, involved intestinal damage, and that more than one disease entity was probably responsible (familial enteropathy [4] and lethal familial protracted diarrhoea [5]).

Davidson et al. [4] described the enteropathy as crypt *hypo*plastic villous atrophy without lamina propria inflammation, indicating that crypt *hyper*plasia (as seen in celiac disease) and an immune-mediated component were not evident. Whilst later studies have questioned the hypoplastic nature of the enteropathy (see below), this observation was taken further and immunohistological criteria were applied to cases of intractable diarrhoea [6, 7]. This approach allowed a division between immune-mediated and epithelial-based diseases, such that disease categories have been clarified [7] and optimisation of treatment options has been proposed [8]. This paper will concentrate on epithelial-based defects and will not consider autoimmune enteropathy and related immune-mediated disorders or therapeutic options, as these are covered elsewhere.

Idiopathic ulcerating enterocolitis of infancy [9, 10] also is not considered, as its features are more like intractable diarrhoea with an immune basis.

To date a small number of discrete diagnoses have been recognised within the heading of congenital enterocyte defects associated with intractable diarrhoea. The level of evidence for placing them in this category is variable, but at the minimum there is an enteropathy and no, or slight, inflammation in the lamina propria. The un-

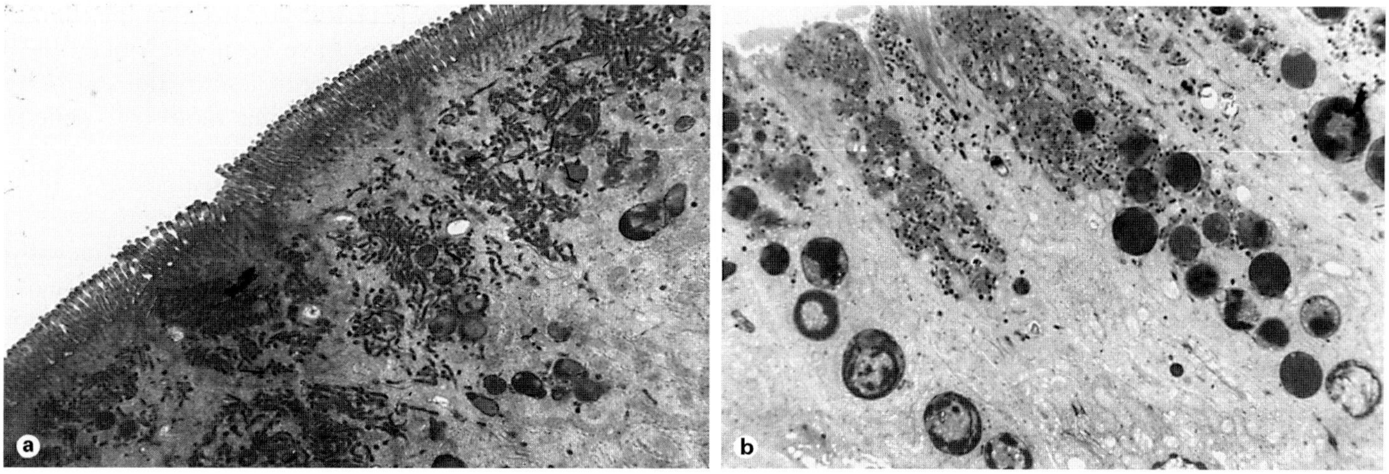

Fig. 2. Microvillous atrophy. Secretory granules in late onset (**a**) and atypical cases (**b**).

derlying abnormalities in these conditions have not been established and work is underway to establish their molecular genetic bases. No gene defects have yet been discovered. Diagnoses include microvillous atrophy or microvillus inclusion disease, tufting enteropathy or epithelial dysplasia, syndromatic diarrhoea or tricho-hepatic-enteric syndrome, idiopathic ulcerating enterocolitis of infancy, and disorders of glycosylation, although idiopathic cases also remain. These are considered in turn below. Several review articles have been published concerning the more common diagnoses within the intractable diarrhoea of infancy syndrome [7, 9–15] and this review will attempt to avoid too much repetition.

Microvillous Atrophy/Microvillus Inclusion Disease

In 1982 at the ESPGHAN annual meeting in Madrid two abstracts were presented that highlighted bizarre findings in the epithelium of infants with intractable diarrhoea. Schmitz et al. [16] coined the term, microvillous atrophy, whereas Goutet et al. [17] referred to Davidson et al. [4] with the descriptive term, familial enteropathy with hypoplastic villous atrophy. Both described the finding of microvillous inclusions within the epithelium, which had been described by Davidson et al. [4] in one of their series of 5 infants; they additionally reported the presence of 'secretory granules' in crypt cells and surface enterocytes [4]. We published 2 more cases of intractable diarrhoea of congenital onset exhibiting an enteropathy with the same distinguishing features (i.e. microvillous inclusions and increased 'secretory granules'; fig. 1, 2) and suggested that these were diagnostic characteristics of the disease [18]. Subsequently Cutz et al. [11] suggested the term, microvillus inclusion disease, in order to highlight the microvillous abnormality.

Clinical Details

The clinical details are well described and accepted to be severe with onset generally occurring in the first week of life [4, 11, 12, 18]. Diarrhoea continues in the absence of enteral feeding and is exacerbated by oral feeding [12]. There appears to be a world-wide distribution of the disease with cases reported from Europe [12], the Middle East [12], Asia [19, 20], and North America [11] including native Americans (Navajo nation) [21]. There are few reports from Africa, although the author has confirmed the diagnosis of microvillous atrophy in a North American of African descent. In developing countries, the severity of the illness may preclude its diagnosis.

The majority of cases present in the first week of life, however in some cases onset of symptoms is after the neonatal period and these have been referred to as 'late onset' microvillous atrophy [12]. The characteristic intestinal morphological abnormalities are present, although with subtle differences (see below), hence the diagnosis. There are few long-term survivors with the disease, although it is considered that 'late onset' cases may have a better prognosis [12]. It is too early to accept this possibility, although in a series of 23 cases, 3 of 5 survivors were 'late onset' [12]. Case 9 in this series is now 23 years old and is doing relatively well on partial parenteral nutrition, but without evidence of improvement in his intestinal abnormality (Ventura A, personal commun.).

As more cases have been diagnosed a wider range of presentation and management courses have been described. These are of interest as they may throw light on the underlying pathogenesis and/or serve as reminders to consider the diagnosis in situations outside accepted dogma, although the majority of cases present as described in the literature [4, 11, 12, 18]. Most cases are not associated with maternal polyhydramnios, however a case was reported recently with polyhydramnios and apparent antenatal bowel obstruction who turned out to have microvillous atrophy [22]. Therefore microvillous atrophy should be considered as part of the differential diagnosis when chloride diarrhoea [23] and Na-H exchange deficiency [24] are possible. Another case of 'late onset' (3 months) and characteristic diagnostic findings spontaneously gained weight at 2 years of age, although diarrhoea continued, and she no longer required parenteral nutrition at 4 years of age [25]. Whilst this case represents an unusual course for this disease, early intestinal transplantation [26] would not have been appropriate for this patient, or perhaps for other 'late onset' cases.

Another interesting event occurred in a case waiting for intestinal and liver transplantation [27]. After a liver biopsy he had a severe intraperitoneal bleed requiring surgery; life-threatening haemorrhagic shock developed with renal failure. Coincidently his diarrhoea decreased, he had no stool for 1 week and then output continued at 10–30 ml/kg/day until transplantation. Enteral feeds produced an increased stool output and there was no change in intestinal morphology. An extreme lowering of hydrostatic pressure, apparently induced a change in the secretory nature of the diarrhoea.

The disease is probably an autosomal recessive trait due to the number of consanguineous parents and the finding of families with affected siblings [12, 28]. Coincident genetic diseases have been described [29, 30], but it is unclear if they represent contiguous gene syndromes or are inherited independently. The high number of consanguineous parents opens the way for molecular genetic studies and the chance of establishing the genetic basis of the disease.

Clinically similar cases of intractable diarrhoea without the diagnostic intestinal features of microvillous atrophy prompted the suggestion that such cases may be related, and are indicative of a spectrum of microvillous disorders [31, 32]. These have been termed intestinal microvillus dystrophy [31]. It is possible that the characteristic diagnostic features have been overlooked [33], and the degree of similarity with microvillous atrophy requires further studies, including molecular genetic analysis.

Pathology

There is an enteropathy with villous atrophy, but without severe crypt hyperplasia, producing a thin mucosa [12]; lamina propria inflammation is absent. This is not hypoplastic villous atrophy [4], as crypt cell numbers are increased [12, 34], as are apoptosis and proliferation [35]. The lack of crypt cell hyperplasia is not due to a limited crypt ability to respond as epidermal growth factor treatment increases intestinal cell proliferation, but without an improvement in clinical state [34]. Epithelial cell death compromises digestion and absorption and is one reason for the diarrhoeal state.

If the small intestine is stained with periodic acid-Schiff (PAS) stain an abnormal accumulation of PAS-positive material is seen in the apical cytoplasm of epithelial cells. In congenital microvillous atrophy this occurs in upper crypt epithelium, whereas in 'late onset' cases the accumulation appears in low villous epithelium, and a normal brush border PAS stain is seen in lower cells [12]. In a third variant, termed 'atypical' microvillous atrophy, the PAS abnormality occurs in the low crypt, and towards the surface epithelium some normal brush border PAS staining is observed [12]. The PAS abnormality suggests that a brush border-destined substance accumulates within the cell rather than being transported to the apical membrane. This distribution parallels the electron microscopy (EM) observation of an increase in 'secretory granules'. The two abnormalities likely represent the same phenomenon [36]. Thus, the secretory granules contain material that is positioned normally in the brush border. EM of the 'granules' showed that they were not discrete granules but made up a vesicular network [36]. The Golgi complex was normal indicating a post-Golgi block in exocytosis. The routine PAS gives the opportunity of retrospective diagnosis [36].

EM has demonstrated the other hall mark of microvillus atrophy, the presence of microvillous lined vacuoles, or inclusions, within the apical cytoplasm of surface epithelial cells (fig. 1), i.e. these occur at a later time in the epithelial cell life cycle than do secretory granules. They can occur as small or large inclusions and occasionally appear as invaginations of the apical membrane or as 'blister-like' profiles with microvilli on one side of the inclusion (fig. 1b). Microvillous inclusions undergo lysosomal digestion and autolysosomal bodies may have microvillous fragments in them. In many cases microvilli may be seen on lateral epithelial cell membranes.

Microvillous inclusions and an increase in secretory granules have been described in both the small and large bowel [18], but not in the stomach; they have not been described in the renal epithelium or in the liver, but they do appear in the gall bladder epithelium.

The brush border is abnormal in this disease, as indicated by the term microvillous atrophy. However, it must be realised that in congenital microvillous atrophy microvilli appear normal in the crypt region and appear variably short or absent on the villus. In 'late onset' cases normal microvilli appear in the low villous region. In 'atypical' microvillous atrophy microvilli are short or absent on upper crypt cells, and they reappear on surface exposed epithelium. These patterns of microvillous appearance parallel the distribution of secretory granules, i.e. once the granules have appeared the microvilli shorten, and if the secretory granules reduce in number then the microvilli reappear [12].

Diagnosis

The diagnosis can be readily made with PAS staining and transmission EM of proximal small intestinal mucosal biopsies. The simplest approach is to perform PAS staining on well-orientated formalin-fixed tissue and look for an accumulation of PAS-positive material in the epithelial apical cytoplasm, usually in the upper crypt or low villous region. If this is found then transmission EM should be performed to determine if microvillous inclusions can be seen. These should be present in surface-located epithelial cells, so orientation is important, and difficulties will arise in a cross-sectionally cut sample.

Various staining techniques have been suggested as diagnostic tools, including alkaline phosphatase [37], carcinoembryonic antigen [38] and CD10 antigen [39], to avoid the requirement for EM which, although important [40], is seen as technically demanding. These techniques can demonstrate the presence of microvillous inclusions, rather than the PAS abnormality. There is a better chance of a definitive diagnosis if both abnormalities are considered and there is a danger of misdiagnosis if only histochemical means are employed as positive staining also may be located in autophagosomes.

Pathogenesis

The disease's pathogenesis is unknown. The presence of microvillous inclusions indicates that there may be a basic disorder of cytoskeletal assembly. However, the finding of normal microvilli in cells in their early stages of development in 'congenital' and 'late onset' cases, and the reappearance of microvilli in 'atypical' cases [12] indicate that this is unlikely. The major microvillous cytoskeletal proteins are present in crypt cell apical cytoplasm providing a source for brush border growth and maintenance [41], and this system may be disturbed leading to premature microvillous construction within the cell (fig. 1a), or inappropriate growth on the lateral cell membrane. Microvillous inclusions may arise by engulfment of apical membrane (fig. 1b) [4, 42]. The uptake of luminal material into microvillous inclusions supports this hypothesis [42]. These possibilities are not notably exclusive.

The prevalence of secretory granules (fig. 2) indicates a defect in exocytosis of brush border destined material. The direct and indirect constitutive pathways of brush border enzymes are intact [43] (although enzyme levels are lowered due to cell damage [12]), implying a defect in an unidentified trafficking route. An early paper reported a brush border myosin deficiency [44] suggesting a defect in actin-myosin interactions responsible for the delivery of membrane associated substances to the brush border [45]. Ameen & Salas [46] in a single case report, have also suggested an apical membrane trafficing defect.

The nature of the secretory granules is unknown. Normally they occupy 2.5% of the apical cell volume, whereas in microvillous atrophy it is 40% [46]. Recent data, demonstrating the presence of acetylated sialic acid and blood group antigens in the secretory granules, indicate they contain glycocalyx-like material, which is blocked from exocytosis [47]. This is supported by the flocculent, fibrillar nature of their content (fig. 1a). The glycocalyx forms a hydrophilic polyanionic gel coat on the cell surface and maintains cell surface charge, protects against physical trauma, and regulates ionic & macromolecular access [48]. A lack of the glycocalyx would have profound consequences on normal cell function and accumulation of cellular debris within the cell may disrupt normal processes. In utero, the intestine is bathed with amniotic fluid of similar osmolality to serum, resulting in no osmotic pressure across the gut. This changes dramatically after birth and the lack of a functional intestinal glycocalyx could explain the rapid onset of symptoms and why most cases of microvillus atrophy could result from the inability to exocytose the glycocalyx.

Tufting Enteropathy/Epithelial Dysplasia

Tufting enteropathy or epithelial dysplasia was described in 3 children by Reifen et al. [50]. Onset of diarrhoea was reported in the neonatal period. One previous case was described by Davidson et al. [4], underlining the variable cause of the intractable diarrhoea in those cases. Feeding dramatically reduced stool volume, and nutritional support allowed a normal growth velocity in 2 cases. The key observation was the presence of an enteropathy exhibiting tufts of closely packed surface enterocytes with rounding of the apical membrane that appeared to be coming away from the epithelium. These were not unique to the condition and were reported in coeliac disease, microvillous atrophy, autoimmune enteropathy and controls, but at a much lower frequency (90 vs. 61–<10%) [50]. Tufting was not seen in the crypt epithelium, there were no distinguishing ultrastructural features, no increase in lamina propria cell infiltration, and the enteropathy persisted despite improvement with nutritional support in 2 cases. This puts this condition into the category of a congenital enterocyte disorder rather than an immunological defect. Similar observations were reported in 6 children [51] with additional data concerning basement membrane abnormalities, i.e. reduced laminin and increased heparan sulphate, but the primary or secondary nature of the abnormalities could not be established. Patey et al. [52] investigated adhesion molecules and found an increased presence of desmoglein, an abnormal distribution of $\alpha_2\beta_1$ integrin along the crypt-villus axis, and an increased presence of desmosomes. They deduced that there were abnormal cell-cell and cell-matrix interactions and that these were involved in the pathogenesis.

It is generally considered to be an autosomal recessive condition. Consanguineous parents and several affected siblings are common [15]. Although Reifen et al. [50] reported normal colons in their cases, further reports have shown the colon to be affected with some crypt abnormalities (branching and pseudocysts) [52]. Diagnosis is not necessarily easy as the prevalence of tufts appears to vary with time and repeat biopsies are required to establish the diagnosis, along with the definite exclusion of microvillous atrophy [15]. In some cases lamina propria inflammation may be present as a secondary event and treatment can allow increased caloric intake [53]. There is some evidence that the condition may resolve with time. Two adults, following 13–15 years of treatment, are now off parenteral nutrition [53], and there has been a report of a successful pregnancy in a woman with tufting enteropathy [54].

Further clarification of this condition awaits molecular genetic analyses. An association between tufting enteropathy and polymalformations has been described [55], but this may be coincidental rather than genetically linked.

Integrin Deficiency

Lachaux et al. [56] recently described an infant presenting with pyloric atresia and intractable diarrhoea. Light microscopy showed extensive severe epithelial cell desquamation from the stomach to the rectum, with only crypt epithelial cells remaining in situ. EM of the gut revealed normal desmosomes with separation between the lamina propria and the basal membrane of enterocytes. This disorder is considered to be related to a congenital deficiency of $\alpha_6\beta_4$ integrin, but of an intestinal isoform, as the cutaneous expression of $\alpha_6\beta_4$ integrin appeared normal. This integrin is defective in epidermolysis bullosa in which gross epidermal shedding occurs. It is likely that there is a mutation within the intestinal $\alpha_6\beta_4$ isoform or a deficiency of a related, immunohistochemically cross-reactive, intestinal integrin.

Syndromatic Diarrhoea

A small number of patients have been described as having syndromatic intractable diarrhoea [57, 58]. Similar cases have been reported previously, falling within the 'tricho-hepato-enteric' syndrome [59–61]. In this syndrome cases are small-for-gestational age, and have intractable diarrhoea starting in the first months of life, liver disease, facial dysmorphism, mental retardation and abnormal hair. Small intestinal morphology is variably abnormal ranging from severe villous atrophy to minor villous shortening. Colitis also has been reported [57]. Consanguineous parents are common [58] and sibs with the syndrome have been described [59, 61] suggesting an autosomal recessive condition. Some cases have evidence of immunodeficiency with poor responses to vaccination and hypogammaglobulinaemia.

Prognosis appears to be variable; some cases have succumbed to infection or liver disease, others require total or partial parenteral nutrition, and one case is on oral feeds [58]. Tolerance to enteral feeds was suggested to be related to the state of the small intestine [58]. The relationship between syndromatic intractable diarrhoea and 'tricho-hepato-enteric' syndrome needs to be evaluated further. The clinical pattern suggests either mutation within several genes, inherited together by linkage disequilibrium, or interference with a higher level of control, such as a patterning gene; as relatively few patterning genes have been implicated in hair development, this may allow a more focused search for candidate mutations [15].

Congenital Disorders of Glycosylation and Protein-Losing Enteropathy

Diarrhoea has been associated variably with congenital disorders of glycosylation and one report described severe intractable diarrhoea at 2 weeks of age as a presenting symptom that persisted on parenteral nutrition with profound hypoalbuminaemia [62]. Neurological symptoms developed, there was no response to mannoses treatment and the patient died at 24 months of age from hepatic insufficiency. The basic defect of glycosylation, beyond a type-1 defect, could not be identified.

Three similar cases with intractable diarrhoea and severe protein-losing enteropathy have been reported [63]. In these cases the small intestinal mucosa appeared histologically normal, but there was an absence of heparan sulphate on the lateral epithelial cell membranes. The link between heparan sulphate, protein-losing enteropathy and inflammation was established recently experimentally [64]. All required total parenteral nutrition, although diarrhoea persisted. No neurological abnormalities or other signs of glycosylation defect syndrome were described, although a case of congenital disorder of glycosylation type 1c with severe hypoalbuminaemia and a similar absence of intestinal epithelial heparan sulphate was reported [65], and patients with type-1b congenital disorders of glycosylation have severe diarrhoea and protein-losing enteropathy [66], so there may be similarities between the various conditions.

Other Causes and Summary

Despite the intensive investigation of cases of intractable diarrhoea many cases remain in which the search for characteristic diagnostic features is elusive. Hopefully, as the genetic basis of diseases with distinguishing features is discovered, light may be thrown on aspects of these idiopathic conditions. Certainly, the dedication of paediatric gastroenterology teams caring for these children with disorders of enterocyte development has brought about avenues of management and discrete diagnoses that have allowed focussed and productive research. Nevertheless, diarrhoeas and enteropathies due to congenital diseases of enterocyte defects often persist despite medical intervention unless the gut is transplanted. The possibilities of resolution of these demanding and severe illnesses must surely wait for successful gene therapies.

References

1 Avery GB, Villavicencio O, Lilly JR, Randolph JG: Intractable diarrhoea in early infancy. Pediatrics 1968;41:712–722.
2 Larcher VF, Shepherd R, Francis DEM, Harries JT: Protracted diarrhoea in infancy. Analysis of 82 cases with particular reference to diagnosis and management. Arch Dis Child 1977;52:597–605.
3 Hyman CJ, Reiter J, Rodnan J, Drash AL: Parenteral and oral alimentation in the treatment of the nonspecific protracted diarrheal syndrome of infancy. J Pediatr 1971;78:17–29.
4 Davidson GP, Cutz E, Hamilton JR, Gall DG: Familial enteropathy: a syndrome of protracted diarrhea from birth, failure to thrive, and hypoplastic villous atrophy. Gastroenterology 1978;75:783–790.
5 Candy DCA, Larcher VF, Cameron DJS, et al: Lethal familial protracted diarrhoea. Arch Dis Child 1981;56:15–23.
6 Cuenod B, Brousse N, Goulet O, et al: Classification of intractable diarrhea in infancy using clinical and immunohistological criteria. Gastroenterology 1990;99:1037–1043.
7 Goulet OJ, Brousse N, Canioni D, Walker-Smith JA, Schmitz J, Phillips AD: Syndrome of intractable diarrhoea with persistent villous atrophy in early childhood: a clinicopathological survey of 47 cases. J Pediatr Gastroenterol Nutr 1998;26:151–161.
8 Goulet O, Ruemmele F, Lacaille F, Colomb V: Irreversible intestinal failure. J Pediatr Gastroenterol Nutr 2004;38:250–269.
9 Sanderson IR, Risdon RA, Walker-Smith JA: Intractable ulcerating enterocolitis of infancy. Arch Dis Child 1991;66:295–299.
10 Thapar N, Shah N, Ramsay AD, Lindley KJ, Milla PJ: Long-term outcome of intractable ulcerating enterocolitis of infancy. J Pediatr Gastroenterol Nutr 2005;40:582–588.
11 Cutz E, Rhoads JM, Drumm B, Sherman PM, Durie PR, Forstner GG: Microvillus inclusion disease: an inherited defect of brush-border assembly and differentiation. N Engl J Med 1989;320:646–651.
12 Phillips AD, Schmitz J: Familial microvillous atrophy: a clinicopathological survey of 23 cases. J Pediatr Gastroenterol Nutr 1992;14:380–396.
13 Cutz E, Sherman PM, Davidson GP: Enteropathies associated with protracted diarrhea of infancy: clinicopathological features, cellular and molecular mechanisms. Pediatr Pathol Lab Med 1997;17:335–368.
14 Sherman PM, Mitchell DJ, Cutz E: Neonatal enteropathies: defining the causes of protracted diarrhea of infancy. J Pediatr Gastroenterol Nutr 2004;38:16–26.

15 Goulet O, Phillips AD: Congenital enteropathy involving intestinal mucosa development; in Walker WA, Goulet O, Kleinman RE, Sanderson IR, Sherman P, Shneider B (eds): Paediatric Gastrointestinal Disease. Burlington, Decker, 2004, pp 922–931.
16 Schmitz J, Ginies JL, Arnaud-Battandier F, et al: Congenital microvillous atrophy: a rare cause of neonatal intractable diarrhoea. Pediatr Res 1982;16:1014.
17 Goutet JM, Boccon-Gibod L, Chatelet F, Ploussard JP, Navarro J, Polonovski Cl: Familial protracted diarrhoea with hypoplastic villous atrophy: report of two cases. Pediatr Res 1982;16:1045.
18 Phillips AD, Jenkins P, Raafat F, Walker-Smith JA: Congenital microvillous atrophy: specific diagnostic features. Arch Dis Child 1985;60:135–140.
19 Beck NS, Chang YS, Kang IS, Park WS, Lee HJ, Suh YL: Microvillus inclusion disease in two Korean infants. J Korean Med Sci 1997; 12:452–456.
20 Kaneko K, Shimizu T, Fujiwara S, Igarashi J, Ohtomo Y, Yamashiro Y: Microvillous inclusion disease in Japan. J Pediatr 1999;135: 400.
21 Pohl JF, Shub MD, Trevelline EE, et al: A cluster of microvillous inclusion disease in the Navajo population. J Pediatr 1999;134:103–106.
22 Kennea N, Norbury R, Anderson G, Tekay A: Congenital microvillous inclusion disease presenting as antenatal bowel obstruction. Ultrasound Obstet Gynecol 2001;17:172–174.
23 Makela S, Kere J, Holmberg C, Hoglund P: SLC26A3 mutations in congenital chloride diarrhea. Hum Mutat 2002;20:425–438.
24 Keller KM, Wirth S, Baumann W, Sule D, Booth IW: Defective jejunal brush border membrane sodium/proton exchange in association with lethal familial protracted diarrhoea. Gut 1990;31:1156–1158.
25 Croft NM, Howatson AG, Ling SC, Nairn L, Evans TJ, Weaver LT: Microvillous inclusion disease: an evolving condition. J Pediatr Gastroenterol Nutr 2000;31:185–189.
26 Ruemmele FM, Jan D, Lacaille F, et al: New perspectives for children with microvillous inclusion disease: early small bowel transplantation. Transplantation 2004;77:1024–1028.
27 Randak C, Langnas AN, Kaufman SS, et al: Pretransplant management and small bowel-liver transplantation in an infant with microvillus inclusion disease. J Pediatr Gastroenterol Nutr 1998;27:333–337.
28 Nathavitharana KA, Green NJ, Raafat F, Booth IW: Siblings with microvillous inclusion disease. Arch Dis Child 1994;71:71–73.
29 Assmann B, Hoffmann GF, Wagner L, et al: Dihydropyrimidinase deficiency and congenital microvillous atrophy: coincidence or genetic relation? J Inherit Metab Dis 1997;20:681–688.
30 Heinz-Erian P, Schmidt H, Le Merrer M, Phillips AD, Kiess W, Hadorn HB: Congenital microvillus atrophy in a girl with autosomal dominant hypochondroplasia. J Pediatr Gastroenterol Nutr 1999;28:203–205.
31 Raafat F, Green NJ, Nathavitharana KA, Booth IW: Intestinal microvillous dystrophy: a variant of microvillous inclusion disease or a new entity? Hum Pathol 1994;25:1243–1248.
32 Mierau GW, Wills EJ, Wyatt-Ashmead J, Hoffenberg EJ, Cutz E: Microvillous inclusion disease: report of a case with atypical features. Ultrastruct Pathol 2001;25:517–521.
33 Weeks DA, Zuppan CW, Malott RL, Mierau GW: Microvillous inclusion disease with abundant vermiform, electron-lucent vesicles. Ultrastruct Pathol 2003;27:337–340.
34 Walker-Smith JA, Phillips AD, Walford N, et al: Intravenous epidermal growth factor/urogastrone increases small intestinal cell proliferation in congenital microvillous atrophy. Lancet 1985;ii:1239–1240.
35 Groisman GM, Sabo E, Meir A, Polak-Charcon S: Enterocyte apoptosis and proliferation are increased in microvillous inclusion disease (familial microvillous atrophy). Hum Pathol 2000;31:1404–1410.
36 Phillips AD, Szafranski M, Man LY, Wall WJ: Periodic acid-Schiff staining abnormality in microvillous atrophy: photometric and ultrastructural studies. J Pediatr Gastroenterol Nutr 2000;30:34–42.
37 Lake BD: Microvillus inclusion disease: specific diagnostic features shown by alkaline phosphatase histochemistry. J Clin Pathol 1988;41:880–882.
38 Groisman GM, Ben-Izhak O, Schwersenz A, Berant M, Fyffe B: The value of polyclonal carcinoembryonic antigen immunostaining in the diagnosis of microvillus inclusion disease. Hum Pathol 1993;24:1232–1237.
39 Groisman GM, Amar M, Livne E: CD10: a valuable tool for the light microscopic diagnosis of microvillous inclusion disease (familial microvillous atrophy). Am J Surg Pathol 2002; 26:902–907.
40 Bell SW, Kerner JA, Sibley RK: Microvillous inclusion disease. The importance of electron microscopy for diagnosis. Am J Surg Pathol 1991;15:1157–1164.
41 Fath KR, Obenauf SD, Burgess DR: Cytoskeletal protein and mRNA accumulation during brush border formation in adult chicken enterocytes. Development 1990;109:449–459.
42 Reinshagen K, Naim HY, Zimmer KP: Autophagocytosis of the apical membrane in microvillus inclusion disease. Gut 2002;51:514–521.
43 Phillips AD, Fransen JAM, Hauri HP, Sterchi E: The constitutive exocytotic pathway in microvillous atrophy. J Pediatr Gastroenterol Nutr 1993;17:239–246.
44 Carruthers L, Phillips AD, Dourmashkin R, Walker-Smith JA: Biochemical abnormality in brush border membrane protein of a patient with congenital microvillous atrophy. J Pediatr Gastroenterol Nutr 1985;4:902–907.
45 Fath KR, Trimbur GM, Burgess DR: Molecular motors are differentially distributed on Golgi membranes from polarized epithelial cells. J Cell Biol 1994;126:661–675.
46 Ameen NA, Salas PJ: Microvillus inclusion disease: a genetic defect affecting apical membrane protein traffic in intestinal epithelium. Traffic 2000;1:76–83.
47 Phillips AD, Brown A, Hicks S, et al: Acetylated sialic acid residues and blood group antigens localise within the epithelium in microvillous atrophy indicating internal accumulation of the glycocalyx. Gut 2004;53:1764–1771.
48 Gupta BL: The relationship of mucoid substances and ion and water transport, with new data on intestinal goblet cells and a model for gastric secretion. Symp Soc Exp Biol 1989;43: 81–110.
49 Gillibrand PN: Changes in the electrolytes, urea and osmolality of the amniotic fluid with advancing pregnancy. J Obstet Gynaecol Br Commonw 1969;76:898–905.
50 Reifen RM, Cutz E, Griffiths AM, Ngan BY, Sherman PM: Tufting enteropathy: a newly recognized clinicopathological entity associated with refractory diarrhea in infants. J Pediatr Gastroenterol Nutr 1994;18:379–385.
51 Goulet O, Kedinger M, Brousse N, et al: Intractable diarrhea of infancy with epithelial and basement membrane abnormalities. J Pediatr 1995;127:212–219.
52 Patey N, Scoazec JY, Cuenod-Jabri B, et al: Distribution of cell adhesion molecules in infants with intestinal epithelial dysplasia (tufting enteropathy). Gastroenterology 1997;113: 833–843.
53 Schaeppi M, Shah NF, Long S, et al: Tufting enteropathy also affects the colon. J Pediatr Gastroenterol Nutr 1999;28:569.
54 Cameron DJ, Barnes GL: Successful pregnancy outcome in tufting enteropathy. J Pediatr Gastroenterol Nutr 2003;36:158.
55 Abely M, Hankard GF, Hugot JP, Cezard JP, Peuchmaur M, Navarro J: Intractable infant diarrhea with epithelial dysplasia associated with polymalformation. J Pediatr Gastroenterol Nutr 1998;27:348–352.
56 Lachaux A, Bouvier R, Loras-Duclaux I, Chappuis JP, Meneguzzi G, Ortonne JP: Isolated deficient alpha6beta4 integrin expression in the gut associated with intractable diarrhea. J Pediatr Gastroenterol Nutr 1999;29:395–401.
57 Girault D, Goulet O, Le Deist F, et al: Intractable infant diarrhea associated with phenotypic abnormalities and immunodeficiency. J Pediatr 1994;125:36–42.
58 Martinez-Vinson C, Goulet O, Berrebi D, et al: Syndromatic diarrhea in children. Report of 8 cases. J Pediatr Gastroenterol Nutr 2005;40: 651.

59 Verloes A, Lombet J, Lambert Y, et al: Tricho-hepato-enteric syndrome: further delineation of a distinct syndrome with neonatal hemochromatosis phenotype, intractable diarrhea, and hair anomalies. Am J Med Genet 1997;68: 391–395.
60 Landers MC, Schroeder TM: Intractable diarrhea of infancy with facial dysmorphism, trichorrhexis nodosa, and cirrhosis. Pediatr Dermatol 2003;20:432–435.
61 Stankler L, Lloyd D, Pollitt RJ, Gray ES, Thom H, Russell G: Unexplained diarrhoea and failure to thrive in 2 siblings with unusual facies and abnormal scalp hair shafts: a new syndrome. Arch Dis Child 1982;57:212–216.
62 Mention K, Michaud L, Dobbelaere D, Guimber D, Gottrand F, Turck D: Neonatal severe intractable diarrhoea as the presenting manifestation of an unclassified congenital disorder of glycosylation (CDG-x). Arch Dis Child Fetal Neonatal Ed 2001;85:F217–F219.
63 Murch SH, Winyard PJ, Koletzko S, et al: Congenital enterocyte heparan sulphate deficiency with massive albumin loss, secretory diarrhoea, and malnutrition. Lancet 1996;347: 1299–1301.
64 Bode L, Eklund EA, Murch S, Freeze HH: Heparan sulfate depletion amplifies TNF-alpha-induced protein leakage in an in vitro model of protein-losing enteropathy. Am J Physiol Gastrointest Liver Physiol 2005;288: G1015–G1023.
65 Westphal V, Murch S, Kim S, et al: Reduced heparan sulfate accumulation in enterocytes contributes to protein-losing enteropathy in a congenital disorder of glycosylation. Am J Pathol 2000;157:1917–1925.
66 Niehues R, Hasilik M, Alton G, et al: Carbohydrate-deficient glycoprotein syndrome type Ib. Phosphomannose isomerase deficiency and mannose therapy. J Clin Invest 1998;101: 1414–1420.

Annales Nestlé

Ann Nestlé 2006;64:25–37
DOI: 10.1159/000086497

Congenital Enteropathy and Intestinal Transplantation

Olivier Goulet

Reference Center for Rare Digestive Diseases, Department of Pediatric Gastroenterology-Hepatology and Nutrition, Hôpital Necker – Enfants Malades, Paris, France

Key Words
Intestinal failure · Citrulline · Congenital enteropathy · Parenteral nutrition · Liver disease · Intestinal transplantation · Liver transplantation · Home parenteral nutrition

Abstract
Intestinal failure (IF) requires the use of parenteral nutrition (PN). Causes of severe protracted IF include short bowel syndrome, severe motility disorders (total or subtotal aganglionosis or chronic intestinal pseudo-obstruction syndrome) and congenital diseases of enterocyte development. Severe liver disease may develop in patients with IF as a consequence of both underlying digestive disease and unadapted PN. Catheter-related sepsis and/or extensive vascular thrombosis may impede the continuation of safe and efficient PN. Thus management of patients with IF requires early recognition of the condition and the analysis of its risk of irreversibility. Timing of referral for intestinal transplantation remains a crucial issue. As a consequence, management should include therapies adapted to each stage of IF based on a multidisciplinary approach in centers involving pediatric gastroenterology, PN expertise, home-PN program, pediatric surgery, liver-intestinal transplantation program.

Intestinal failure (IF) is a condition of severe intestinal malabsorption requiring parenteral nutrition (PN). Congenital enteropathies that impair the intestinal mucosa lead to irreversible IF. The risk of complications of permanent PN is high, thus raising the possible need of intestinal transplantation (ITx).

Definition of Intestinal Failure

'Intestinal failure' is defined as the critical reduction of functional gut mass below the minimal amount necessary for adequate digestion and absorption to satisfy body nutrient and fluid requirements for health maintenance in adults or growth in children. However, this definition is not accepted uniformly. Some suggest that IF is better defined in terms of fecal energy losses rather than residual bowel length in patients with short bowel syndrome [1]. Another approach is to evaluate the degree of IF according to the amount of PN required for maintenance in adults and growth in children. Beside anatomic and nutritional criteria for defining IF, a biological marker of gut functional mass has been proposed recently [2]. Citrulline is a nonessential amino acid that is produced mostly by enterocytes [3]. Plasma citrulline levels may be measured easily reflecting the loss of functional mass in patients with short bowel syndrome (SBS) and in patients

KARGER

Fax +41 61 306 12 34
E-Mail karger@karger.ch
www.karger.com

Accessible online at:
www.karger.com/ane

Olivier Goulet, Reference Center for Rare Digestive Diseases
Department of Pediatric Gastroenterology-Hepatology and Nutrition
Hôpital Necker – Enfants Malades, 149 Rue de Sèvres
FR–75743 Paris Cedex 15 (France)
Tel. +33 1 44 49 44 11, Fax +33 1 44 49 25 01, E Mail olivier.goulet@nck.ap-hop-paris.fr

with various degrees of villous atrophy or experiencing intestinal graft rejection with villous atrophy [4]. In a recent study involving short bowel syndrome pediatric patients treated with recombinant human growth hormone, plasma citrulline levels increased significantly following treatment [5]. The current criteria for defining IF remain the inability to preserve growth in children without permanent dependence on PN.

Causes of Intestinal Failure

The natural history of IF in children is variable and influenced largely by the underlying disorder responsible for the loss of intestinal function. The most common type of IF is secondary to gastrointestinal infection. However, children with such acute IF are expected to recover completely with appropriate treatment. Nonetheless, post-enteritis protracted diarrhea remains a leading cause of IF in developing countries [6]. In developed countries, IF is dominated by congenital or early onset of severe and permanent disease requiring protracted or indefinite PN. Historically, SBS was one of the first recognized causes of protracted IF [7]. However, with the increasing and successful use of long-term PN during the last three decades, several other causes of IF emerged, e.g. severe extensive motility disorders including subtotal aganglionosis, chronic intestinal pseudo-obstruction syndrome and congenital diseases of enterocyte development [8].

Congenital Enteropathy Causing Intestinal Failure

An attempt to classify intractable diarrhea of infancy (IDI) with the degree of villous atrophy was proposed on the basis of immunohistological criteria that emphasize the role of activated T cells in the intestinal mucosa [9]. A multicenter survey from ESPGHAN collected cases of IDI and villous atrophy with precisely defined light microscopic characteristics that allowed the categorization of several types of IDI [10]. The first one was characterized by a mononuclear cell infiltration of the lamina propria and considered to be associated with activated T cells. The second histological pattern included early onset of severe diarrhea with villous atrophy without mononuclear cell infiltration of the lamina propria and specific histological abnormalities involving the epithelium. To date, several types of primary epithelial abnormalities inducing IDI have been identified. The first described was microvillous atrophy (MVA) or microvillous inclusion disease and more recently tufting enteropathy or intestinal epithelial dysplasia (IED) [11]. Some small for gestational age patients present with phenotypic abnormalities that correspond to IDI [12].

Microvillous Atrophy

In 1978, Davidson et al. [13] reported 5 infants with severe, persistent diarrhea beginning in the newborn period, in whom light microscopy revealed crypt hypoplastic villous atrophy. Electron microscopic examination of small intestinal biopsies from 3 of the patients showed severe brush border abnormalities and increased liposome-like bodies, and in 1, intracytoplasmic cysts with a brush border architecture. Children were also reported with characteristic cytoplasmic inclusions of the brush border membrane [14]. From these clinical and histological descriptions, MVA was established as a distinct disease within the syndrome of IDI. In its typical form MVA is a congenital disorder of intestinal epithelial cells that presents initially as neonatal intractable diarrhea [14].

Clinical Expression

In general, infants develop severe watery diarrhea within the first days after birth. Stool volumes may be as high as 250–300 ml/kg body weight/day and fecal electrolyte concentrations are similar to those of the small intestinal fluid. This disorder is particularly life-threatening since massive diarrhea leads to rapid dehydration, electrolyte imbalances, and subsequent metabolic decompensation within a few hours. Severe watery diarrhea persists despite bowel rest. Differential diagnoses may include congenital chloride diarrhea and sodium malabsorption diarrhea that can be distinguished easily from MVA by assessment of blood and stool electrolytes [15–16]. In contrast, the clinical presentation of MVA also may be very atypical with a full and distended small bowel and colon mimicking a pseudo-occlusion sydrome. The most common onset of diarrhea in MVA is within the first few days (early-onset or congenital form). However, in a few patients onset of diarrhea may be delayed (first month) and less severe (late-onset form).

Histopathological Analyses

Diagnosis may be made easily from a light microscopic examination of a duodenal or jejunal biopsy specimens. On hematoxylin-eosin staining, the mucosa appears flattened with hypoplastic villous atrophy. Highly character-

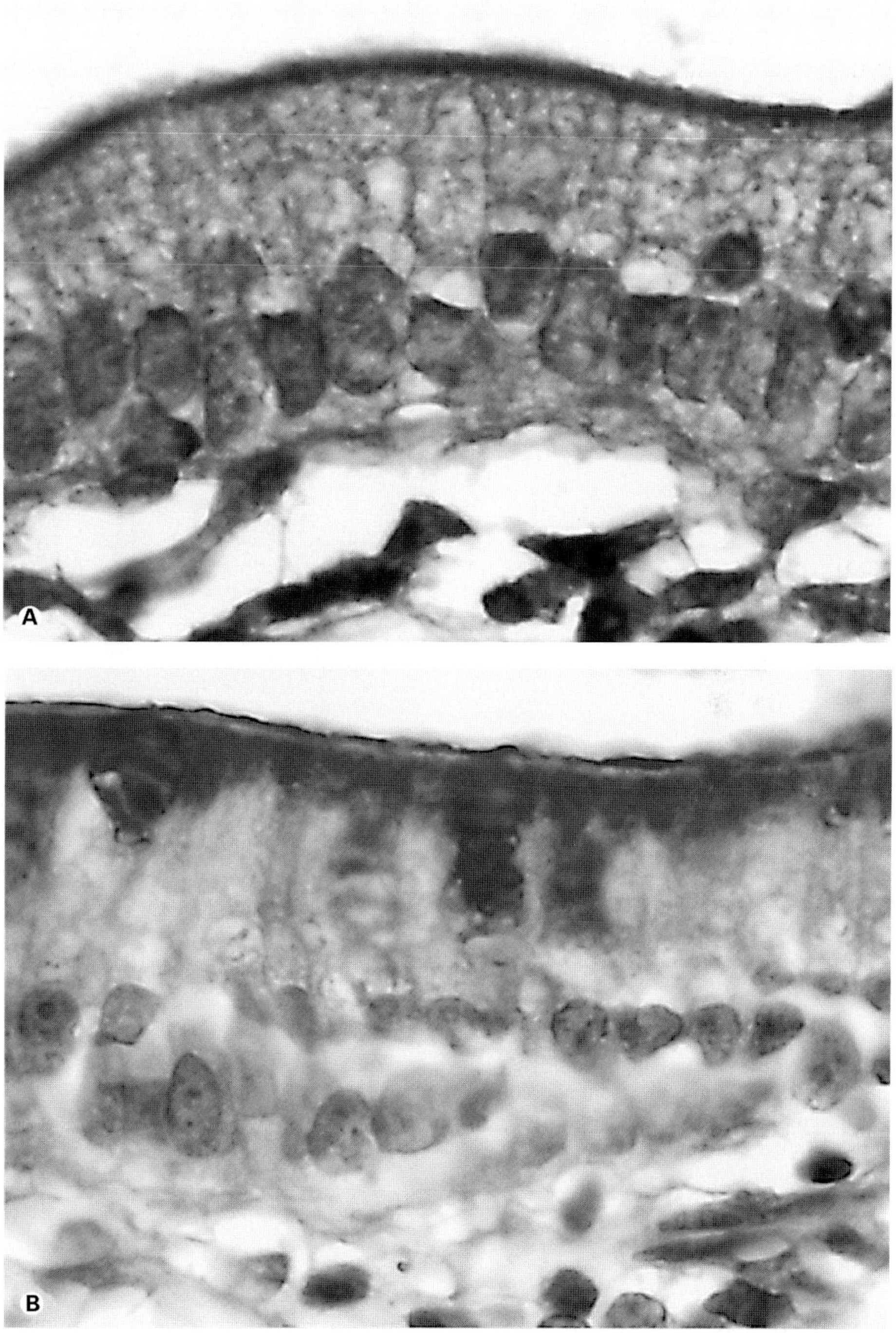

Fig. 1. Periodic acid-Schiff (PAS) staining. **A** Normal mucosa, normal PAS, brush border staining. **B** Abnormal accumulation of PAS, positive material in the apical cytoplasm of epithelial cells in microvillous inclusion disease.

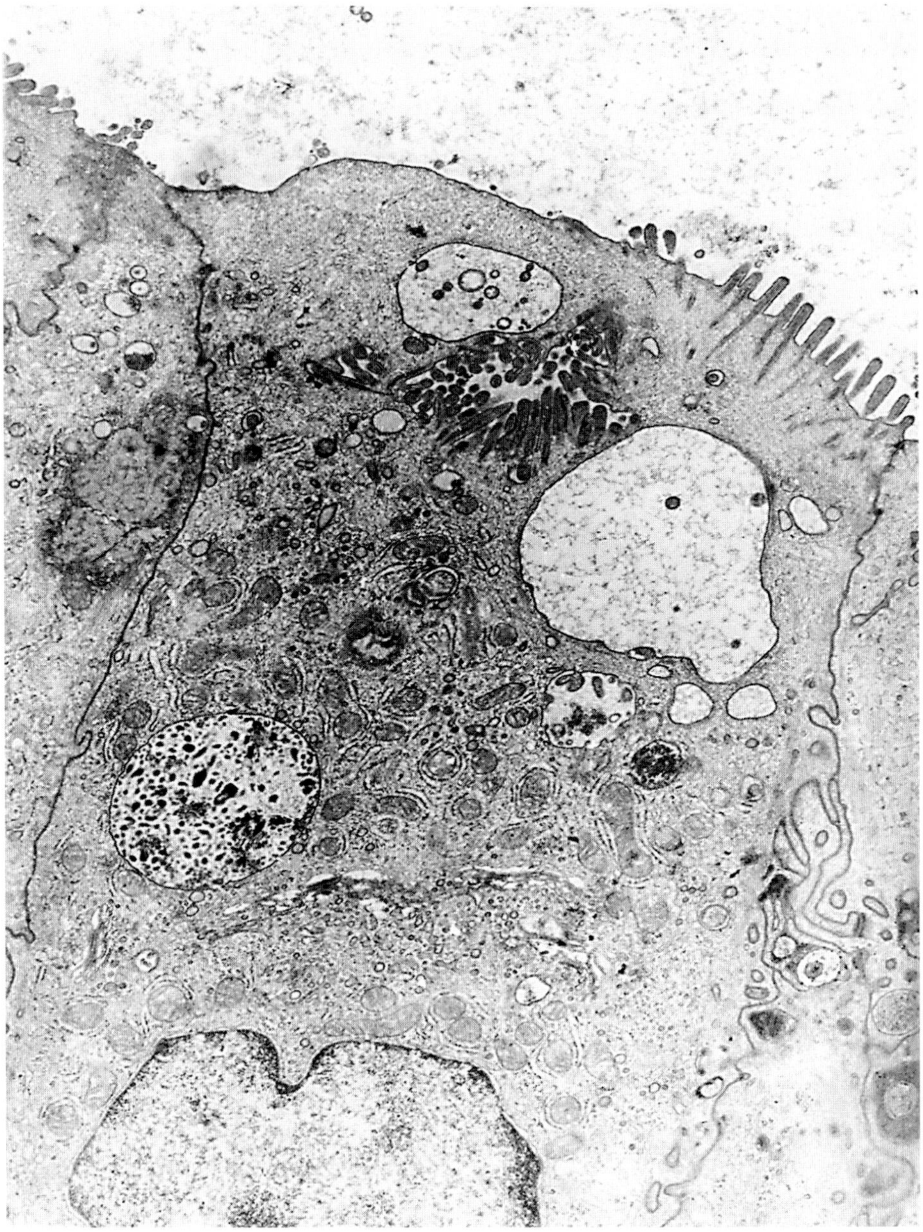

Fig. 2. Microvillous inclusion disease. Electron microscopy of a jejunal biopsy specimen. The brush border is almost absent. The cytoplasm contains a microvillous inclusion.

istic for this disorder is the accumulation of periodic acid-Schiff (PAS)-positive secretory granules within the apical cytoplasm of enterocytes [17, 18] (fig. 1). On the ultrastructural level, rare or absent microvilli and cytoplasm inclusions of microvilli of enterocytes are seen. These anatomical changes define this entity [19]. A new valuable tool for the light microscopic diagnosis of MVA was proposed recently [20, 21]. CD-10 is a membrane-associated neutral peptidase, shown to have a linear brush border staining pattern in the normal small intestine. In contrast to this surface staining in different conditions (normal intestine, celiac disease, autoimmune enteropathy, and allergy), all MVA cases demonstrate prominent intracytoplasmic CD-10 immunoreactivity in surface enterocytes [20]. Similar results were obtained with PAS, polyclonal carcinoembryonic antigen and alkaline phosphatase, three stains known to show cytoplasmic staining of surface enterocytes in MVA [22]. On electron microscopy, surface epithelial cells show absent or grossly abnormal microvilli, and numerous vesicular bodies of various sizes, and characteristic microvillous inclusions (fig. 2). Crypt cells are morphologically almost normal. They do not contain increased numbers of apical vesicles and vesicular bodies. Microvillous inclusions and increased secretory granules are also present in the large bowel epithelium. This is particularly important because this tissue is more easily accessible for biopsy, especially in early infancy.

Pathophysiology and Mode of Transmission

A defect in the membrane trafficking of immature and/or differentiating enterocytes also was discussed as an etiopathogenic mechanism in MVA [19, 22]. A direct functional consequence of this membrane defect is complete IF. It has been speculated that this disease is associated with a disorder of the enterocyte cytoskeleton. The cytoskeleton produces an abnormal assembly of microvilli. Intestinal microvillous dystrophy was reported to be a hypothetic variant of MVA [22]. The underlying pathogenesis of MVA, however, remains unclear. When analyzing the turnover of sucrase-isomaltase, as a representative brush border protein, there is clear evidence that direct and indirect constitutive pathways are intact in MVA [19]. Since in both congenital and late onset MVA, microvilli appear to be near normal in regions where secretory granules first accumulate, a defect in microvillous biosynthesis is not likely to be the basis of the disease. Recently, by investigating the secretory granules, Phillips et al. [23] suggested that MVA involves a defect in the exocytosis of the glycocalyx that might impair normal cell functions.

Considering the number of cases with affected siblings and the frequency of consanguinity among patients, this disease appears to be transmitted as an autosomal recessive trait [24]. To date no candidate gene has been identified, but MVA was reported in a girl with autosomal dominant hypochondroplasia [25]. The gene defect of this hypochondroplasia was localized recently to chromosome region 4p16.3. This might help to elucidate the genetic basis of MVAs.

Long-Term Outcome

The largest multicenter survey of 23 MVA patients [14] revealed an extremely reduced life expectance, with a 1-year survival rate of less than 25%. Most children died of septic complications, liver failure or metabolic decompensation. Few cases of MVA, especially the late-onset form, and those with limited stool outputs may survive with only partial PN. Treatment with corticosteroids, colostrum or epidermal growth factor has not been successful, but octreotide was used with partial success in 1 patient [14]. Contrary to the initial outcome before the 1980s, PN now allows most infants and children to survive. However, complications related to inadequate PN limit long-term survival. In addition, without evidence of an associated renal disease, some of these infants and children present with chronic hydro-electrolytic imbalances and acidosis with subsequent impaired growth. Some others, because of repeated dehydration episodes associated with inappropriate phosphocalcic intakes, present with nephrocalcinosis. Finally, even with adequate long-term PN and normal growth, high and uncomfortable stool outputs persist and often require daily fluid and electrolyte replacements with the high risk of severe dehydration. Thus, ITx may be the only definitive treatment for this rare intestinal disease.

Several cases of successful transplantation for MVA were reported [26–29]. Transplantation involved isolated intestine [26] or combined transplants with the liver [27, 28]. Whether or not the colon should be transplanted with the small bowel remains controversial. We recently reported patients with early-onset congenital MVA [29]. Two patients died before they could be put on a waiting list for small bowel transplantation, 1 patient is still awaiting small bowel transplantation. We have performed cadaveric ITx in 7 patients aged between 3 and 11 years using tacrolimus, steroids and IL-2 blockers. Three ITx were performed and 4 associated with the liver. Right colon transplantation was performed in 5 cases (2 isolated ITx). Six patients (86%) have survived with a median follow-up of 3 (range 1–8) years. Complete weaning from PN was achieved in all patients. For the first time ITx alone or in combination with the liver offered MVA children a long-term perspective [29, 30].

Intestinal Epithelial Dysplasia or Tufting Enteropathy

Three cases of neonatal severe diarrhea with abnormal epithelial pictures were reported by Reifen et al. [31] under the name 'tufting enteropathy'. We identified 9 cases of severe neonatal diarrhea which were clearly different from MVA [11]. Further studies in these patients showed that intestinal epithelial dysplasia (IED) is a constitutive epithelial disorder involving both the small intestine and colon [32]. In our experience IED seems frequent in patients of Arabic origin, and in the Middle-East and North Africa. A main characteristic of this disease is its clinical and histological heterogeneity and its association with malformations or other epithelial diseases.

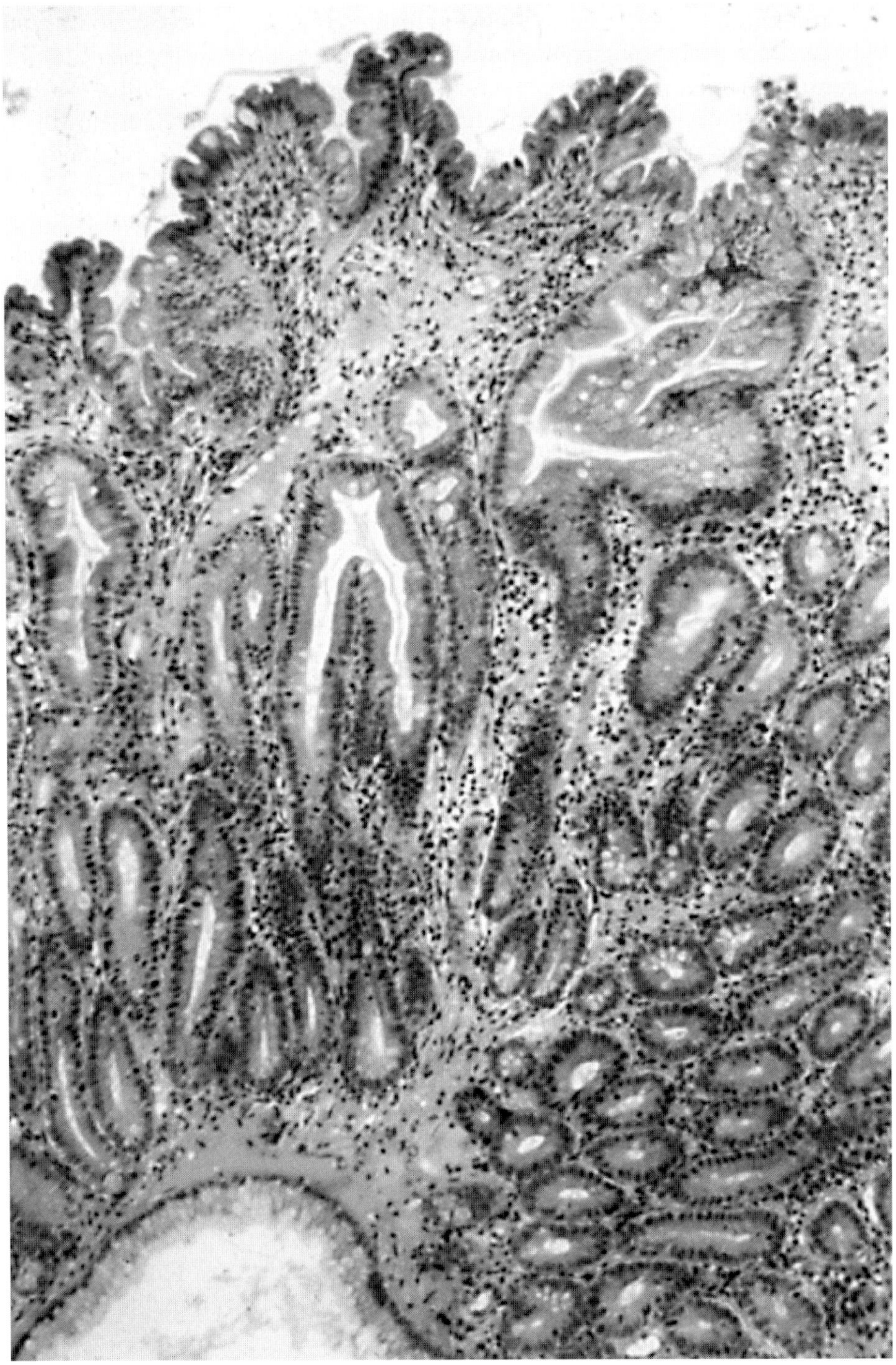

Fig. 3. Intestinal epithelial dysplasia. Partial villous atrophy with crypt hyperplasia and/or pseudocystic crypt appearance, branching pictures and disorganization of surface epithelium.

Clinical Expression

Typically, patients present during the first weeks of life with severe diarrhea. Most have consanguineous parents and/or an affected sibling. Some affected family members died during the first months of life with severe diarrhea of unknown origin. Most of the time, diarrhea persisted despite bowel rest but mortality was less than that observed with MVA. Attempts to use continuous enteral feeding with a protein hydrolysate or amino acids worsened diarrhea. Newborns rapidly fail to thrive and develop severe protein energy malnutrition.

Histological Presentation

Villous atrophy is present but variable in severity. In its typical form, abnormalities are localized mainly to the epithelium and include a disorganization of surface enterocytes with focal crowding resembling tufts (fig. 3). These characteristic 'tufts' of extruding epithelium, first described by Reifen et al. [31], are seen towards the villous tip, and may affect up to 70% of the villi. The tufting process is not limited to the small intestine but also involves the colonic mucosa [11]. This picture also can be observed in the crypt epithelium and, in addition, crypts often have an abnormal aspect with dilatation such as pseudocysts and abnormal regeneration with branching [11]. Study of the basement membrane components demonstrated abnormal laminin and heparan sulfate proteoglycan deposition at that level compared to biopsy specimens from patients with celiac disease or autoimmune enteropathy [11]. Relative to controls, there was faint and irregular laminin deposition at the epithelial lamina propria interface while heparan sulfate proteoglycan deposits were large and lamellar suggestive of the abnormal development of the basement membrane. These may be the origin of the epithelial abnormalities. On the other hand, we observed an increased immunohistochemical expression of desmoglein in IED, and ultrastructural changes in desmosomes that were increased in length and number [32] (fig. 4).

IED is suspected most often after elimination of MVA on PAS stained slides. Its final diagnosis is made after repeated intestinal biopsies which change from subnormal in early life (only nonspecific villous atrophy with or without monocellular cell infiltration of the lamina propria) to the characteristic tufts. Another difficulty is related to the infiltration of the lamina propria by T cells. T cell infiltrates support the diagnosis of an immune-related enteropathy, as previously described especially when tufts are missing. One can speculate that defective cell adhesion increases intestinal permeability with a subsequent inflammatory reaction. Murch et al. [33] described this type of lesion in infants with epithelial dysplasia.

Associated Disorders

Several cases of IED were reported as being associated with specific phenotypic abnormalities, e.g. Dubowitz syndrome or malformation syndrome [34, 35]. An association between congenital IDI and choanal atresia was reported recently in 4 children [34]. We have observed malformations including rectal or esophageal atresia and recently reported a nonspecific punctiform keratitis involving about 60% of patients [36]. This keratitis is very intriguing since it is also an epithelial disease that might help to elucidate the molecular mechanisms of intestinal epithelial disease. The fact that some children have no ophthalmologic symptoms illustrates the likely heterogeneity of the disease.

Interestingly, Lachaux et al. [37] recently reported the case of a newborn presenting with pyloric atresia and intractable diarrhea. Light microscopic examination showed extensive desquamation from the fundus to the rectum with only a few epithelial cells remaining at the crypt bases. Electron microscopy of the gut epithelium revealed normal desmosomes but a cleavage located between the lamina propria and the basal pole of the enterocytes. This initial description was related to a congenital deficiency of the $\alpha 6\beta 4$ integrin known to be defective in epidermolysis bullosa.

Pathophysiology and Mode of Transmission

IED was shown to be associated with an abnormal basement membrane compared to those from biopsy specimens from patients with celiac disease or autoimmune enteropathy [11]. Basement membrane molecules are involved in epithelial mesenchymal cell interactions, which are instrumental in intestinal development and differentiation [38]. Alterations suggestive of abnormal cell–cell and cell–matrix interactions were seen in patients with IED without any evidence for abnormalities in epithelial cell polarization and proliferation [32]. Alterations included an abnormal distribution of adhesion molecules, the $\alpha 2\beta 1$ integrin along the crypt–villous axis. The $\alpha 2\beta 1$ integrin is involved in the interaction of epithelial cells with various basement membrane components, such as laminin and collagen. Pathophysiological mechanisms resulting in an increased immunohistochemical expression of desmoglein, and the ultrastructural changes in desmosomes remain unclear [32]. A mouse with a loss of function change in the

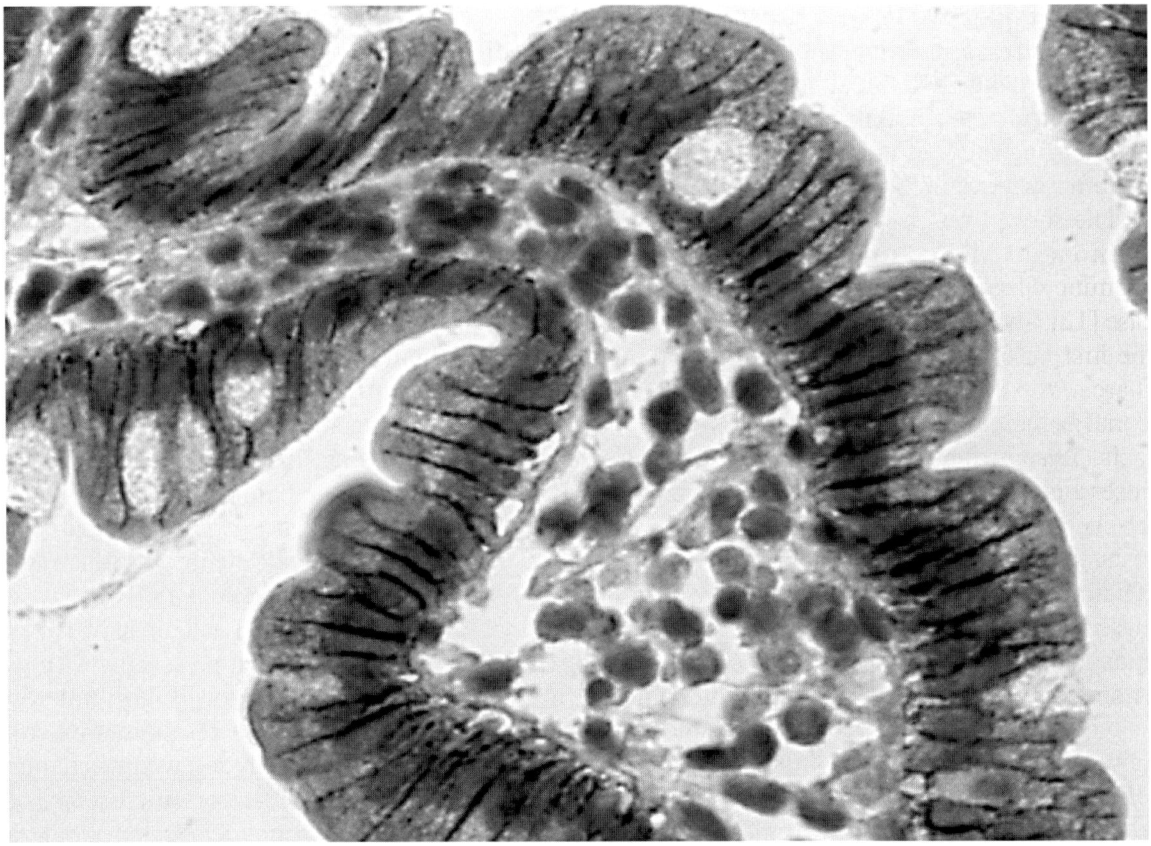

Fig. 4. Intestinal epithelial dysplasia. Increased expression of desmoglein staining of the tight junction in a patient with intestinal epithelial dysplasia.

gene encoding the transcription factor Elf3 has morphologic features resembling epithelial dysplasia in infants [39]. In this mouse model, there is abnormal morphogenesis of the villi and progenitor crypt cells appear normal. The enterocytes in Elf3-deficient mice produce low levels of the transforming growth factor-β type-2 receptor that induces the differentiation of immature intestinal epithelia. Currently, in human infants, the primary or secondary nature of the observed modifications remains to be determined. The presence of tufts may provide important clues. Tufts correspond to non-apoptotic epithelial cells at the villous tips that are no longer in contact with the basement membrane. Although speculative, a defect in normal enterocyte apoptosis at the end of their lifespan or an altered cell–cell contact may be responsible for this effect. The primary or secondary nature of the formation of tufts remains to be determined.

To date the genetic origin of this disorder is suspected from the clear association of parental consanguinity and/or affected siblings. These features suggest an autosomal recessive transmission. The gene involved in this congenital inherited autosomal recessive disease is not yet identified. This enteropathy appears more common than MVA, especially in the Middle-East population.

Outcome

Neonatal diarrhea that resists all treatments requires permanent PN. However, it seems that some infants develop milder phenotype than others [40]. Because of partial residual intestinal function and the limited amount of stool output, some patients need only partial long-term PN with 3–4 times weekly infusions. However, careful monitoring should be performed to avoid progressive growth retardation. In most patients, the severity of intestinal malabsorption and diarrhea makes them totally dependent on daily long-term PN with a subsequent risk of complications. IED can be another indication for ITx [41, 42].

Other Congenital Enteropathies

The so-called 'phenotypic diarrhea', which is an IDI syndrome associated with phenotypic abnormalities and immune deficiency, also is a rare, recently reported disease [12]. Affected patients present with diarrhea within the first 6 months of life (<1 month in most cases) and share several clinical features. They are small for gestational age and have an abnormal phenotype [12]. All have facial dysmorphism with prominent foreheads, broad noses and hypertelorism. They have a distinct hair abnormality, tricorrhexis nodosa, in which the hair is woolly, difficult to manage, easily pulled out and poorly pigmented. These features also are seen in children of Middle-East origin. Among the congenital forms of hair dysplasia, trichorrhexis nodosa is very common and can be present in several pathologic conditions [43, 44]. These patients also have defective antibody responses despite normal serum immunoglobulin levels, and defective antigen-specific skin tests despite positive proliferative responses in vitro [12]. Small bowel biopsy specimens of patients with syndromatic diarrhea show moderate or severe villous atrophy with inconstant mononuclear cell infiltrates of the lamina propria and the absence of epithelial abnormalities. Histologically, there are no specific abnormalities. The prognosis of this type of IDI is poor since most patients die between the ages of 2 and 5 years. Some suffer the early onset of liver disease [12]. The cause of this diarrhea is unknown and the relationships among low birth weight, dysmorphism, severe diarrhea, trichorrhexis and immune deficiency are unclear.

Management of Intestinal Failure

Long-Term Parenteral Nutrition

Whether in hospital or at home, long-term PN exposes the patient to several complications including catheter-related sepsis and thrombosis, liver and bone disease [45]. Daily catheter care and prevention of septic complications are essential [46]. Liver function tests should be performed on a regular basis because of the risk of cholestasis and liver injury. Ultrasonography aiming to look for sludge or cholelithiasis should be repeated at least twice a year in patients with gall bladders. In addition, bone mineralization should be examined using DEXA, phosphorus and calcium status should be assessed, and diets should be managed to prevent PN-related bone disease.

Factors and Management of Liver Disease

Liver disease is the most frequent and the most severe complication in IF patients. The expression 'PN-related liver disease' should be replaced by 'IF-related liver disease'. Indeed, the most important factors inducing cholestasis and end-stage liver disease are related to impaired intestinal function and bacterial overgrowth. Liver injury is aggravated further by inadequate PN.

The main factors related to liver disease may be listed as follows:

(1) Disruption of the enterohepatic cycle (ileal disease or resection) [47, 48]

(2) Intestinal stasis with subsequent intraluminal bacterial overgrowth and/or translocation (endotoxinemia) [49]

(3) Recurrent catheter-related sepsis [50, 51]

(4) Prematurity [51]

(5) Inadequate macronutrient intake such as continuous PN infusion with excessive glucose intake leading to hyperinsulinism and subsequent steatosis [52] and inadequate amino acid supply [49]

(6) Excessive intake of long-chain polyunsaturated fatty acids with subsequent lipoperoxidation [53, 54] and high content of phytosterols from soybean oil-based emulsions [55]

(7) Aluminum, iron and/or chromium overloads [56–58]

Premature and/or small for gestational age infants with severe necrotizing enterocolitis are at especially high risk of developing liver disease and early end-stage liver failure because of the combination of prematurity, subocclusion, Gram-negative sepsis, protracted bowel rest, continuous instead of cyclic PN infusion, and repeated catheter-related sepsis.

Prevention or resolution of liver injury may be possible by:

(1) Stimulating enterobiliary axis by ensuring the ingestion of long-chain triglycerides or breast milk, or by injection of cholecystokinin analogs [59]

(2) Suppressing the intraluminal bacterial overgrowth caused by intestinal stasis by giving metronidazole [60] and/or performing tapering enteroplasty

(3) Using ursodesoxycholic acid (30 mg/kg/day) to decrease liver injury [61]

(4) Avoiding catheter-related sepsis by appropriate daily care of the line [50, 51]

(5) Adapting PN intake by:

(a) Limiting glucose intake to reduce hepatic fat accumulation [62, 63], and

(b) Using the appropriate type and amount of intravenous fat emulsion to provide essential fatty acids, reducing glucose load and limiting peroxidation [53–55]. The recent development of olive oil-based fat emulsions may reduce peroxidation [54]. The daily administration of intravenous lipid should not exceed 2–2.5 g/kg

(6) Controlling the lipid supply and rate of delivery and/or stopping intravenous lipids as soon as thrombocytopenia, hyperbilirubinemia and/or jaundice appear [53]

(7) Using new pediatric adapted amino acid solutions that provide appropriate amino acids plus taurine [49]

(8) Performing cyclic PN that reduces hyperinsulinism and liver steatosis [64]

(9) Adapting iron intake and decreasing the aluminum content of the PN solutions [65]

With appropriate care and prevention, liver disease may be delayed or even avoided and the patient may be maintained in a nutritional and general condition offering better prognosis when isolated small bowel transplantation is required for irreversible IF.

Intestinal Transplantation

Whatever the cause of protracted or irreversible IF, long-term PN is the mainstay of therapy. Home PN allows infants and children to grow in the best psychological environment [66, 67]. The irreversibility of IF has to be demonstrated before ITx is considered.

When ITx becomes the indicated therapeutic option, extensive multidisciplinary discussions among transplant surgeons and pediatric gastroenterologists are mandatory. Assessments and decisions are based on the occurrence of complications listed during the workshop held at the International Symposium on Small Bowel Transplantation in Miami, September 2003. These criteria are similar to those reported in the position paper of the American Society of Transplantation [68] and continue to be debated, especially those that relate to vascular thrombosis and sepsis:

(1) Liver disease (bilirubin levels >3 mg/dl, splenomegaly, thrombocytopenia, gastroesophageal varices, coagulopathy, stomal bleeding, hepatic fibrosis, or cirrhosis)

(2) Thrombosis of major venous accesses (>2 thromboses in subclavian, jugular, or femoral veins). In our practice 1 access left in the superior vena cava bed

(3) Recurrent catheter-related sepsis (2 episodes of systemic sepsis secondary to line infection per year, 1 episode of line-related fungemia, septic shock, or acute respiratory distress syndrome)

(4) Underlying disease causing uncontrollable water electrolyte losses and frequent severe acute dehydration

These criteria are guidelines, not formal recommendations. They must be balanced with the risks of ITx.

Contraindications to ITx do not differ from those pertaining to other solid organs. Due to the risks of ITx, especially in cases of poor recipient conditions at the time of transplantation and the donor pool size, the concept that the patient must have the potential to derive an obvious benefit from the procedure must remain paramount.

Other contraindications include congenital or acquired neurological disabilities, life-threatening extra-digestive illnesses, congenital or acquired immune disorders, non-resectable malignancy, and insufficient vascular patency to guarantee easy central venous access for up to 6 months after ITx.

Type of Transplantation

Patients with irreversible IF and end-stage liver disease (liver cirrhosis) are clearly candidates for life-saving procedures such as combined liver-small bowel transplantation (LITx). Patients with severe hepatic fibrosis are more difficult to manage. Repeated liver biopsies within 6–12 months and careful assessments of portal hypertension are necessary. In addition, it is difficult to assess the amount of functional liver tissue necessary to withstand the insult of portal diversion during the transplantation procedure. Children with severe advanced and progressive hepatic fibrosis are usually candidates for LITx. However, some PN-dependent patients with advanced liver dysfunction may experience functional and biochemical liver recovery that occurs parallel to autologous gut salvage. Several consecutive cases of severe cholestasis recovered totally after discontinuation of intravenous lipid administration [69]. Histology is not always predictive of functional liver recovery [70]. Once cirrhosis has been established, however, survival at 1 year is only 20–30% [71].

Timing of Referral for Intestinal Transplantation

Factors impacting the survival of children with IF referred for ITx are well known including: age <1 year; surgical disease; bridging fibrosis or cirrhosis; bilirubin levels

>3 mg/dl, and thrombocytopenia [71]. It is well established that patients referred to intensive care centers for LITx are debilitated, have multiple complications and prolonged stays. The UNOS report indicates that mortality of patients on ITx waiting lists is higher than on other transplantation waiting lists [72]. It may explain the low patient and graft survival rates reported in various studies [73]. The Intestinal Transplant Registry confirmed that transplantations performed in patients waiting at home versus waiting in hospital have a better 1-year survival (74 vs. 59%; $p < 0.00001$) [73]. The trend to transplant proportionately more patients who are waiting at home was a major factor contributing to the recently improved graft and patient survival rates [73].

Few centers manage all the stages of IF from onset to ITx, including the home PN program. A marked discrepancy was reported in clinical status between children referred for ITx from centers with and without nutritional care teams [74]. Long-term management of IF has become a very important concern as suggested by recently published studies [75]. A national or international network might provide data on IF on which the needs for health care should be based [76] and make it possible to optimize management, upgrade the medical approach and to promote basic and applied research in the field. Indeed, appropriate management of IF requires reference centers using therapeutic strategies that are based on a multidisciplinary approach that involves pediatric gastroenterologists, nutritionists, pediatric surgeons, specialized nurses, dieticians, social workers and psychologists. This integrated approach should be adapted to each type and stage of IF including home PN and a transplantation program.

Conclusion

Early management of IF in reference centers by a multidisciplinary group is the key to the timely recognition of IF and its reversal, improved outcomes, and timely ITx. As recently stressed by a Working Group report of Pediatric Gastroenterology and Nutrition, research is needed in all fields of adaptation after small bowel resection and to identify the genes involved in congenital enteropathy or intestinal pseudo-obstruction syndrome [77]. It is also mandatory to assess the respective costs of long-term home PN and ITx and target the best option for maximizing the quality of life of affected children and their families.

References

1 Nordgarrd I, Hansen BS, Mortensen PB: Importance of colonic support for energy absorption as small-bowel failure proceeds. Am J Clin Nutr 1996;64:222–231.

2 Crenn P, Coudray-Lucas C, Thuillier F, Cynober L, Messing B: Postabsorptive plasma citrulline concentration is a marker of absorptive enterocyte mass and intestinal failure in humans. Gastroenterology 2000;119:1496–1505.

3 Crenn P, Vahedi K, Lavergne-Slove A, Cynober L, Matuchansky C, Messing B: Plasma citrulline: A marker of enterocyte mass in villous atrophy-associated small bowel disease. Gastroenterology 2003;124:1210–1219.

4 Pappas PA, Saudubray JM, Tzakis AG, et al: Serum citrulline and rejection in small bowel transplantation: a preliminary report. Transplantation 2001;72:1212–1216.

5 Dabbas-Tyan M, Colomb V, Rosilio M, Landais P, Ricour C, Goulet O: Evaluation of the effect of recombinant human growth hormone (rhGH) treatment of children with short bowel syndrome. J Pediatr Gastroenterol Nutr 2000; 31:S165–S166.

6 Walker-Smith JA: Diarrhoeal disease: current concepts and future challenges. Malnutrition and infection. Trans R Soc Trop Med Hyg 1993;87(suppl 3):13–15.

7 Goulet O, Révillon Y, Jan D, et al: Neonatal short bowel syndrome. J Pediatr 1991;119:18–23.

8 Goulet O, Ruemmele F, Lacaille F, Colomb V: Irreversible intestinal failure. J Pediatr Gastroenterol Nutr 2004;38:250–269.

9 Cuenod B, Brousse N, Goulet O, et al: Classification of intractable diarrhea in infancy using clinical and immunohistological criteria. Gastroenterology 1990;99:1037–1043.

10 Goulet O, Brousse N, Canioni D, et al: Syndrome of intractable diarrhoea with persistent villous atrophy in early childhood: A clinicopathological survey of 47 cases. J Pediatr Gastroenterol Nutr 1998;26:151–161.

11 Goulet O, Kedinger M, Brousse N, et al: Intractable diarrhea of infancy: a new entity with epithelial and basement membrane abnormalities. J Pediatr 1995;127:212–219.

12 Giraut D, Goulet O, Ledeist F, et al: Intractable diarrhea syndrome associated with phenotypic abnormalities and immune deficiency. J Pediatr 1994;125:36–42.

13 Davidson GP, Cutz E, Hamilton JR, Gall DG: Familial enteropathy: a syndrome of protracted diarrhea from birth, failure to thrive, and hypoplastic villous atrophy. Gastroenterology 1978;75:783–790.

14 Phillips AD, Schmitz J: Familial microvillous atrophy: A clinicopathological survey of 23 cases. J Pediatr Gastroenterol Nutr 1992;14: 380–396.

15 Holmberg C: Congenital chloride diarrhea. Clin Gastroenterol 1980;3:583–602.

16 Booth IW, Stange G, Murer H, Fenton TR, Milla PJ: Defective jejunal brush-border Na+/H+ exchange: a cause of congenital secretory diarrhoea. Lancet 1985;i:1066–1069.

17 Phillips AD, Jenkins P, Raafat F, Walker-Smith JA: Congenital microvillous atrophy: specific diagnostic features. Arch Dis Child 1985;60:135–140.

18 Phillips AD, Szfranski M, Man L-Y, Wall W: Periodic acid Schiff staining abnormality in microvillous atrophy: photometric and ultrastructural studies. J Pediatr Gastroenterol Nutr 2000;30:34–42.

19 Phillips A, Fransen J, Hauri HP, Sterchi E: The constitutive exocytotic pathway in microvillous atrophy. J Pediatr Gastroenterol Nutr 1993;17:239–246.
20 Groisman GM, Amar M, Livne E: CD10: A valuable tool for the light microscopic diagnosis of microvillous inclusion disease (familial microvillous atrophy). Am J Surg Pathol 2002; 26:902–907.
21 Youssef N, Canioni D, Ruemmele F, et al: CD-10 expression in microvillous inclusion disease (abstract). J Pediatr Gastroenterol Nutr 2003; 36:563.
22 Raafat F, Green NJ, Nathavitharana KA, Booth IW: Intestinal microvillous dystrophy: a variant of microvillous inclusion disease or a new entity? Hum Pathol 1994;25:1243–1248.
23 Phillips AD, Brown A, Hicks S, Schuller S, Murch SH, Walker-Smith JA, Swallow DM: Acetylated sialic acid residues and blood group antigens localise within the epithelium in microvillous atrophy indicating internal accumulation of the glycocalyx. Gut 2004;53:1764–1771.
24 Nathavitharana KA, Green NJ, Raafat F, Booth IW: Siblings with microvillous inclusion disease. Arch Dis Child 1994;71:71–73.
25 Heinz-Erian P, Schmidt H, Le Merrer M, et al: Congenital microvillous atrophy in a girl with autosomal dominant hypochondroplasia. J Pediatr Gastroenterol Nutr 1999;28:203–205.
26 Oliva MM, Perman JA, Saavedra JM, et al: Successful intestinal transplantation for microvillous inclusion disease. Gastroenterology 1994;106:771–774.
27 Herzog D, Atkinson P, Grant D, et al: Combined bowel-liver transplantation in an infant with microvillous inclusion disease. J Pediatr Gastroenterol Nutr 1996;22:405–408.
28 Randak C, Langnas AN, Kaufman SS, et al: Pretransplant management and small bowel-liver transplantation in an infant with microvillous inclusion disease. J Pediatr Gastroenterol Nutr 1998;27:333–337.
29 Ruemmele FM, Jan D, Lacaille F, et al: New perspectives for children with microvillous inclusion disease: early small bowel transplantation. Transplantation 2004;77:1024–1028.
30 Croft NM, Howatson AG, Ling SC, et al: Microvillous inclusion disease: an evolving condition. J Pediatr Gastroenterol Nutr 2000;31: 185–189.
31 Reifen RM, Cutz E, Griffiths AM, Ngan BY, Sherman PM: Tufting enteropathy: a newly recognized clinicopathological entity associated with refractory diarrhea in infants. J Pediatr Gastroenterol Nutr 1994;18:379–385.
32 Patey N, Scoazec JY, Cuenod-Jabri B, et al: Distribution of cell adhesion molecules in infants with intestinal epithelial dysplasia (tufting enteropathy). Gastroenterology 1997;113: 833–843.
33 Murch S, Graham A, Vermault A, et al: Functionally significant secondary inflammation occurs in a primary epithelial enteropathy. J Pediatr Gastroenterol Nutr 1997;24:467.
34 Krantz M, Jansson U, Rectors S, Ryd W, Kristiansson B: Hereditary intractable diarrhea with choanal atresia. A new familial syndrome. J Pediatr Gastroenterol Nutr 1997;24:470.
35 Abely M, Fromont Hankard G, et al: Intractable infant diarrhea with epithelial dysplasia associated with polymalformation. J Pediatr Gastroenterol Nutr 1998;27:348–352.
36 Djeddi D, Verkarre V, Talbotec C, et al: Tufting enteropathy and associated disorders (abstract). J Pediatr Gastroenterol Nutr 2002;34: 446.
37 Lachaux A, Bouvier R, Loras I, et al: Isolated deficient $\alpha 6\beta 4$ integrin expression in the gut associated with intractable diarrhoea. J Pediatr Gastroenterol Nutr 1999;29:395–401.
38 Simon-Assmann P, Kedinger M: Heterotypic cellular cooperation in gut morphogenesis and differentiation. Cell Biol 1993;4:221–230.
39 Ayn NG, Waring P, Ristevski S, et al: Inactivation of the transcription factor Elf3 in mice results in dysmorphogenesis and altered differentiation of intestinal epithelium. Gastroenterology 2002;122:1455–1466.
40 Cameron DJS, Barnes GL: Successful pregnancy outcome in tufting enteropathy. J Pediatr Gastroenterol Nutr 2003;36:158.
41 Lacaille F, Cuenod B, Colomb V, et al: Successful combined liver and small bowel transplantation in a child with epithelial dysplasia. J Pediatr Gastroenterol Nutr 1998;27:230–233.
42 Paramesh AS, Fishbein T, Tschernia A, et al: Isolated small bowel transplantation for tufting enteropathy. J Pediatr Gastroenterol Nutr 2003;36:138–140.
43 Itin PH, Pittelkow MR: Trichothiodystrophy: review of sulfur-deficient brittle hair syndromes and association with the ectodermal dysplasia. J Am Acad Dermatol 1990;22:705–717.
44 Verloes A, Lombet J, Lambert Y, et al: Tricho-hepato-enteric syndrome: further delineation of a distinct syndrome with neonatal hemochromatosis phenotype, intractable diarrhea, and hair anomalies. Am J Med Genet 1997;68: 391–395.
45 Shulman RJ, Phillips S: Parenteral nutrition in infants and children. J Pediatr Gastroenterol Nutr 2003;36:587–607.
46 Colomb V, Fabeiro M, Dabbas M, Goulet O, Merckx J, Ricour C: Central venous catheter-related infections in children on long-term home parenteral nutrition: incidence and risk factors. Clin Nutr 2000;19:355–359.
47 Colomb V, Goulet O, Rambaud C, et al: Long term parenteral nutrition in children: liver and gallbladder disease. Transplant Proc 1992;24: 1054–1055.
48 Moss RL, Das JB, Raffensperger JG: Total parenteral nutrition-associated cholestasis: clinical and histopathological correlation. J Pediatr Surg 1993;28:1270–1275.
49 Forchielli ML, Walker WA: Nutritional factors contributing to the development of cholestasis during total parenteral nutrition. Dev Pediatr 2003;50:245–267.
50 Colomb V, Jobert-Giraud A, Lacaille F, Goulet O, Fournet JC, Ricour C: Role of lipid emulsions in cholestasis associated with long-term parenteral nutrition in children. J Parenter Enteral Nutr 2000;24:345–350.
51 Moseley RH: Sepsis-associated cholestasis. Gastroenterology 1997;112:302–305.
52 Lienhardt A, Rakotoambinina B, Colomb V, et al: Insulin secretion and sensitivity in children on cyclic total parenteral nutrition. J Parenter Enteral Nutr 1998;22:382–386.
53 Belli DC, Fournier LA, Lepage G, et al: Total parenteral nutrition-associated cholestasis in rats: comparison of different amino acid mixtures. J Parenter Enteral Nutr 1987;11:67–73.
54 Goulet O, de Potter S, Antebi H, et al: Long-term efficacy and safety of a new olive oil-based intravenous fat emulsion in pediatric patients: a double-blind randomized study. Am J Clin Nutr 1999;70:338–345.
55 Clayton PT, Whitfield P, Iyer K: The role of phytosterols in the pathogenesis of liver complications of pediatric parenteral nutrition. Nutrition 1998;14:158–164.
56 Popinska K, Kierkus J, Lyszkowska M, et al: Aluminum contamination of parenteral nutrition additives, amino acid solutions, and lipid emulsions. Nutrition 1999;15:683–686.
57 Ben Hariz M, Goulet O, De Potter S, et al: Iron overload in children receiving prolonged parenteral nutrition. J Pediatr 1993;123:238–241.
58 Moukarzel A, Song MK, Buchman AL, et al: Excessive chromium intake in children receiving total parenteral nutrition. Lancet 1992; 339:385–388.
59 Ling PR, Sheikh M, Boyce P, et al: Cholecystokinin (CCK) secretion in patients with severe short bowel syndrome (SSBS). Dig Dis Sci 2001;46:859–864.
60 Capron JP, Gineston JL, Herve MA: Metronidazole in prevention of cholestasis associated with total parenteral nutrition. Lancet 1983;i:446–447.
61 Heubi JE, Wiechmann DA, Creutzinger V, et al: Tauroursodeoxycholic acid (TUDCA) in the prevention of total parenteral nutrition-associated liver disease. J Pediatr 2002;141:237–242.
62 Bresson JL, Narcy P, Putet G, et al: Energy substrate utilization in infants receiving total parenteral nutrition with different glucose to fat ratios. Pediatr Res 1989;25:645–648.
63 Kaufman SS: Prevention of parenteral nutrition-associated liver disease in children. Pediatr Transplant 2002;6:37–42.
64 MacFie J: Cyclic parenteral nutrition. Nutrition 1997;13:46–48.
65 Advenier E, Landry C, Colomb V, et al: Aluminum contamination of parenteral nutrition and aluminum loading in children on long-term parenteral nutrition. J Pediatr Gastroenterol Nutr 2003;36:448–453.
66 Colomb V, Goulet O, Ricour C: Home enteral and parenteral nutrition: Baillieres Clin Gastroenterol 1998;122:877–894.

67 Scolapio JS: A review of the trends in the use of enteral and parenteral nutrition support. J Clin Gastroenterol 2004;38:403–407.
68 Kaufman S, Atkinson JB, Bianchi A, Goulet O, Grant D, Langnas A, et al: Indications for pediatric intestinal transplantation: A position paper of the American Society of Transplantation. Pediatr Transplant 2001;5:80–87.
69 Colomb V, Jobert-Giraud A, Lacaille F, Goulet O, Fournet JC, Ricour C: Role of lipid emulsions in cholestasis associated with long-term parenteral nutrition in children. JPEN J Parenter Enteral Nutr 2000;24:345–350.
70 Iyer K, Horslen S, Torres C, et al: Histology is not predictive of functional liver recovery in parenteral-nutrition associated liver dysfunction (abstract). Pediatr Transplant 2003;7:69.
71 Bueno J, Ohwada S, Kocoshis S, et al: Factors impacting the survival of children with intestinal failure referred for intestinal transplantation. J Pediatr Surg 1999;34:27–33.
72 Fryer J, Pellar S, Ormond D, Koffron A, Abecassis M: Mortality in candidates waiting for combined liver-intestine transplants exceeds that for other candidates waiting for liver transplants. Liver Transplant 2003;9:748–753.
73 Grant D, Abu-Elmagd K, Reyes J, Tzakis A, Langnas A, Fishbein T, Goulet O: Farmer D, on the behalf of the Intestine Transplant Registry: 2003 report of the intestine transplant registry: a new era has dawned. Ann Surg 2005; 241:607–613.
74 Beath SV, Booth IW, Murphy MS, et al: Nutritional care and candidates for small bowel transplantation. Arch Dis Child 1995;73:348–350.
75 Fishbein TM, Schiano T, LeLeiko N, et al: An integrated approach to intestinal failure. Results of a new program with total parenteral nutrition, bowel rehabilitation, and transplantation. J Gastrointest Surg 2002;6:554–562.
76 Guarino A, De Marco G, Italian National Network for Pediatric Intestinal Failure: Natural history of intestinal failure, investigated through a national network-based approach. J Pediatr Gastroenterol Nutr 2003;37:136–141.
77 Kocoshis SA, Beath S, Booth IW, Oliva GA, Goulet O, Kaufman SS, Lai HS, Luque C, Ohtsuka Y: Intestinal failure and small bowel transplantation, including clinical nutrition: Working Group report of the second World Congress of Pediatric Gastroenterology, Hepatology and Nutrition. J Pediatr Gastroenterol Nutr 2004;39(suppl 2):S655–S661.

Annales Nestlé

Ann Nestlé 2006;64:39–47
DOI: 10.1159/000086498

Persistent Diarrhea in Developing Countries

Zulfiqar A. Bhutta

Department of Paediatrics and Child Health, Aga Khan University, Karachi, Pakistan

Key Words

Diarrhea, persistent · Micronutrient deficiency · Malnutrition · Immune deficiency · Therapy, inappropriate, acute diarrhea

Abstract

Globally diarrheal diseases account for almost a fifth of all deaths of children under 5 years, with an estimated 2.2 million deaths annually. Of these deaths, a significant proportion are related to episodes of persistent diarrhea (PD; defined as diarrhea of >14 days with growth faltering). PD has been shown to identify children with a substantially increased diarrheal burden. These account for 36–54% of all diarrhea-related deaths. Although the exact pathogenesis of PD remains unclear, most episodes are related to prior acute infectious diarrhea with prolongation of the most recent episode. This may be related to several host factors such as preexisting undernutrition, micronutrient deficiency, immune deficiency and inappropriate therapy of the most recent acute diarrheal episode. The common final event appears to be prolonged intestinal mucosal injury and ineffective repair. In contrast to post-infectious PD, some infants may have severe intractable diarrhea due to a variety of disorders, many of which have a hereditary basis. These now form the dominant type of prolonged diarrhea in developed countries. The management of PD depends upon close attention to nutritional rehabilitation and early recognition of complications. Although a variety of pathogens have been associated with PD, there is little role for oral antimicrobial therapy in the routine treatment of PD. However, attention to rehydration, appropriate screening and treatment of systemic infections and enteral nutrition rehabilitation with easily digestible diets are critical in managing such children, frequently in ambulatory settings. Administration of zinc and vitamin A may shorten the duration of PD and also help reduce recurrences. However, the most important preventive strategies for PD are exclusive breastfeeding in the first 6 months of life, continued breast- feeding for 2 years with appropriate complementary feeding and optimal management of acute diarrheal episodes.

Introduction

Despite considerable advances in the understanding and management of diarrheal disorders in childhood, globally these still account for a large proportion (20%) of childhood deaths, with an estimated 2.2 million deaths [1]. In a global estimate of the burden of diarrheal disorders in 1980 the World Health Organization calculated that there were over 700 million episodes of diarrhea annually in children under 5 years of age in developing countries (excluding China), with approximately 4.6 million deaths [2]. More recent reviews of studies published

KARGER

Fax +41 61 306 12 34
E-Mail karger@karger.ch
www.karger.com

0517–8606/06/0641–0039$23.50/0

Accessible online at:
www.karger.com/ane

Zulfiqar Ahmed Bhutta
Department of Paediatrics and Child Health
Aga Khan University, PO Box 3500, Stadium Road
Karachi 74800 (Pakistan)
Tel. +92 21 4930051/ext. 4724, Fax +92 21 4934294, E-Mail zulfiqar.bhutta@aku.edu

in the last 10 years indicate that although global mortality may have been reduced, the overall incidence remains unchanged at about 3.2 episodes per child year [2–5]. However, it is important to point out that the amount of information available from good quality epidemiological surveys between these time periods also varied significantly and relatively few studies were conducted recently. The previous survey undertaken in 1993 included 276 studies conducted in 60 countries [3], whereas the 2003 review had data from only 31 studies conducted in 20 countries [5].

It is recognized that most diarrheal disorders form a continuum, with the majority of cases resolving within the first week of illness. However, a smaller proportion of diarrheal illnesses fail to resolve and persist for longer than 2 weeks. Persistent diarrhea (PD) is defined as episodes that began acutely but last for at least 14 days [6]. These criteria identify children with a substantially increased diarrheal burden and an increased rate of diarrhea-related deaths. Such episodes were recognized to account for 3 to 20% of all diarrheal episodes in children under 5 years of age [7]. In several large community-based studies of diarrhea [8, 9] it has been shown that PD is directly responsible for between 36 and 54% of all diarrhea-related deaths. It has, however, been pointed out that such differences in mortality between different regions may be related to environmental characteristics and differences in the utilization of health care and oral rehydration therapy [10]. Although PD accounted for only 5% of all diarrheal episodes in a large prospective study of diarrhea in north India, the case fatality rate for PD was 14% in comparison with 0.7% for episodes of shorter duration [11].

It is important to recognize that most cases of PD in developing countries represent post-infectious diarrhea. The majority of cases of diarrhea in developing countries are of acute onset and are shorter than 1 week in duration. However, a group of children develop episodes of longer duration, some lasting longer than 14 days [12]. Although the aforementioned division of diarrheal episodes into acute and PD may be arbitrary, this operational definition identifies children with significantly increased diarrheal burdens. In a prospective study in northeastern Brazil, Lima et al. [13] demonstrated that all children with a heavy diarrheal burden (defined as >16% of total days spent with diarrhea) had at least one episode of PD during a 1-year study period. Similar observations by Moy et al. [14] in a rural cohort of 204 children in Zimbabwe indicated that although PD accounted for only 6% of all diarrheal episodes, these included 22% of the total days of diarrhea recorded in this study and that these children also had higher rates of diarrheal relapse at follow-up. Thus, children with PD may not represent a distinct subgroup but form part of a continuum in susceptibility to diarrhea. Many children (especially infants and toddlers) in developing countries may have frequent recurrent episodes of acute diarrhea. While few individual episodes may persist beyond 14 days, frequent recurrences of acute diarrheal episodes do result in nutritional compromise and may predispose these children to develop PD.

In contrast to PD in developing countries, cases of prolonged diarrhea among young children in developed countries may fall under the category of intractable diarrhea of infancy. These cases are defined as diarrhea lasting for at least 2 weeks where at least 50% of the daily fluid requirement may need to be provided intravenously. Many of these disorders have a genetic basis and may also be seen in developing countries, although their prevalence is greatly overshadowed by those of post-infectious PD.

Review Methods

A recent working group on PD reviewed the information and actions needed at the level of pediatricians, training institutions and professional societies [15]. However, the review did not elaborate upon recent epidemiological trends, and interventions needed in public health systems. This current review will present an overview of the current status of epidemiological information and evidence gaps for clinical care as well as public health interventions.

In order to assess recently available information and trends, we reviewed all the available information on diarrhea epidemiology and PD over the last 15 years (1990–2004) in electronic medical (PubMed/Medline, Extra Med, Pop Line) and social science libraries. Other search terms such as 'chronic diarrhea', 'prolonged diarrhea' and 'intractable diarrhea' also were used to search for published relevant reports. In addition a manual search of relevant monographs and WHO/UNICEF materials also was conducted to access recent information on PD and management strategies targeting children. The available studies were then classified into those addressing epidemiology or burden estimates, pathogenesis, management strategies at either facility or community settings and available randomized controlled trials. We also evaluated studies of PD that related to the HIV status of populations and related pathogens such as cryptosporidium, *Giardia lamblia,* etc.

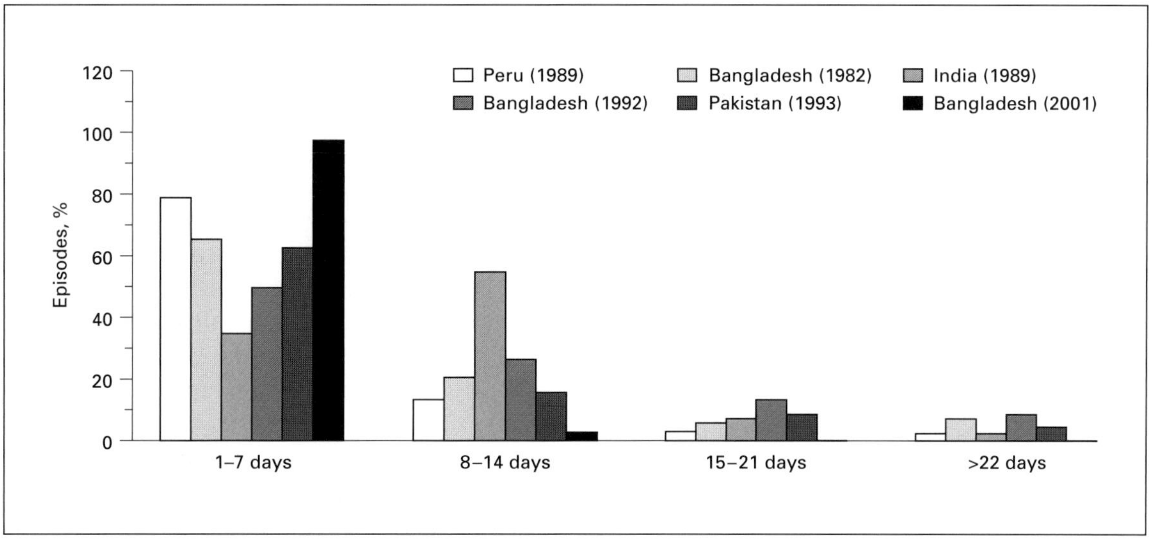

Fig. 1. Incidence of childhood diarrhea in community settings [11, 17–20].

It was evident that the bulk of the epidemiological information on the relationship of acute diarrheal episodes to PD was derived from studies undertaken over a decade ago. There was a remarkable paucity of recent data on this subject, especially from non-HIV endemic areas. However, it was evident from studies in HIV endemic areas that chronic enteropathy and PD was increasingly recognized as common manifestations of advancing HIV infection and AIDS [16].

There is little evidence overall that the true global incidence of PD has decreased. Figure 1 indicates the duration of diarrhea from several community-based studies in developing countries [11, 17–20]. Although recent data from community-based studies on diarrhea are relatively sparse, the overall rates of PD from community settings appeared remarkably constant over the period between 1980 and 1992. A recent community-based study from Bangladesh [20] indicates that PD accounted for less than 0.5% of all cases of diarrhea in an urban community setting, and it is difficult to generalize about trends in the reduction of the burden of PD. There is a clear need to review the previously estimated proportions of acute diarrheal episodes that become prolonged.

The HIV/AIDS epidemic in Africa has resulted in a change in the usual etiological patterns of diarrhea. Prolonged episodes associated with infections due to relatively rare organisms such as cryptosporidium are more common.

Pathogenesis of PD

Prolonged diarrhea in childhood also may arise from a large number of conditions, many of them non-infectious. The most common of these disorders are: cow/soy milk protein intolerance (in infants <6 months old, often with blood-tinged stools); celiac disease (gluten-sensitive enteropathy), and cystic fibrosis (creatorrhea and steatorrhea secondary to pancreatic insufficiency). In other instances, toddler's diarrhea also may be seen in relatively well-nourished infants.

However, globally the most important underlying trigger for PD is an acute diarrheal episode due to an enteric infection and the consequences thereof. There have been several studies on pathogens causing PD in developing countries but few have pinpointed a major causative organism. Although it may appear that PD is a consequence of poor management of acute infectious diarrhea, some pathogens are isolated with greater frequency from children with PD. Table 1 indicates the various organisms that have been associated with PD among children from different parts of the world.

Globally almost a quarter of all diarrhea deaths are associated with dysentery, a large proportion caused by *Shigella* organisms. In a recent study from Bangladesh [21], PD was seen in 23% of children with shigellosis and *Shigella* infections were significantly associated with an increased risk of PD (age-adjusted relative risk 1.83; 95% confidence interval 1.19–2.81). Infection by multiple an-

Table 1. Pathogens associated with prolonged and persistent diarrhea

Bacteria	Enteroaggregative *Escherichia coli* Enteropathogenic *Escherichia coli* *Campylobacter* *Salmonella enteritides* *Shigella* species *Clostridium difficile* *Arcobacter butzleri* *Klebsiella* species
Parasites	*Giardia lamblia* *Blastocystis hominis*[1] *Cryptosporidium* spp.[1] *Entamoeba histolytica* *Cyclospora cayetanensis*[1]
Viruses	Human astrovirus 3 Enterovirus Picobernaviruses

[1] Especially associated with HIV infections/AIDS.

Table 2. Etiology of intractable diarrhea of infancy

1	Congenital chloride diarrhea
2	Microvillus inclusion disease
3	Epithelial dysplasia or Tufting enteropathy
4	Autoimmune enteropathy
5	Food allergy
6	Chronic intestinal pseudo-obstruction/Hirschsprung's disease
7	Intestinal lymphangiectasia
8	Abeta-lipoproteinemia
9	Eosinophilic enteropathy
10	Intestinal neurodysplasia
11	Congenital enzymatic deficiency (congenital glucose-galactose malabsorption, sucrase-isomaltase deficiency, etc.)
12	Trichorrhexis nodosa, facial dysmorphism, immune deficiency and cirrhosis

tibiotic-resistant *Shigella* isolates (age-adjusted relative risk 3.76; 95% confidence interval 1.51–9.36) and occurrence of shigellosis during infancy were observed to be risk factors for initiation of *Shigella* diarrhea persistence. However, 88% of the persistent shigellosis episodes occurred in older children, 50% were associated with non-dysenteric shigellosis and 79% were caused by *Shigella* species other than *Shigella dysenteriae.* Other organisms may similarly affect mucosal inflammation. An additional pathogenic mechanism underlying entero-aggregative *Escherichia coli* infections may include the induction of IL-8 and mucosal inflammation.

In contrast to PD, there is much greater understanding of the mucosal absorptive and transport mechanisms underlying intractable diarrhea in developed countries. Table 2 indicates some of the major causes of intractable diarrhea of infancy.

It is now recognized that mutations of the Cl^-/HCO_3^- exchanger of the ileocolonic apical membrane (solute carrier family 26, member 3 gene [SLC26A3, alias CLD or DRA]) result in the net secretion of chloride by the intestine and a clinical syndrome recognized as congenital chloride-losing diarrhea [22]. Similarly it is recognized that congenital glucose/galactose malabsorption is the result of a genetic defect resulting in a reduction or absence of functional sodium-coupled glucose transporter SGLT1 at the enterocyte cell surface [23], and a number of genotype/phenotype relationships have been recognized [24]. Congenital sucrase-isomaltase deficiency (CSID) also presents with osmotic diarrhea following the introduction of sucrose/complex starches into the weaning diet. Molecular and cell biological studies have defined the pathogenesis of CSID extremely well demonstrating that CSID appears to be a result both of defective synthesis and glycoprotein processing [25].

In contrast, detailed studies from developing countries of mucosal abnormalities and factors underlying mucosal abnormalities in PD are woefully rare and none have explored the molecular mechanisms of prolonged intestinal injury. The most striking example of the critical role that the immune system plays in the pathogenesis of PD is the relationship of HIV/AIDS with PD. This is exemplified by a host of studies linking PD with cryptosporidiosis [26] and other parasitic infections in Africa and Asia. Although these observations suggest that immune deficiency may be related to the risk of prolonged diarrhea [27], there also has been much interest in the possibility that a transient immune deficiency also may be a marker of concomitant micronutrient deficiency [28, 29].

An additional factor underlying poor intestinal repair may include key micronutrient deficiencies that can influence this process. From initial studies indicating the potential benefit of zinc supplementation on reducing the risk of prolonged diarrhea [30], recent meta-analyses of zinc supplementation in diarrheal illnesses indicate a significant reduction in the duration and severity of diarrheal illnesses [31]. Thus zinc deficiency may significantly contribute to the prolongation of mucosal injury and delayed intestinal repair mechanisms. The benefits of

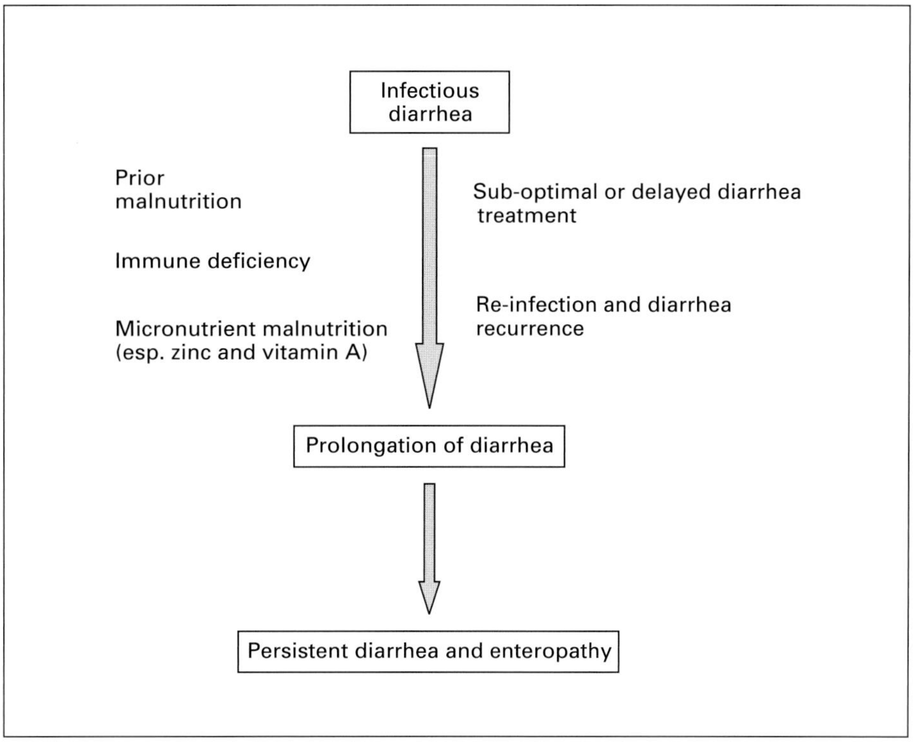

Fig. 2. Pathway to prolonged and persistent diarrhea.

zinc in reducing mortality from childhood diarrhea have led to its inclusion in the current recommendations for diarrhea management by WHO/UNICEF [32]. However, very little is known about the mechanisms of action of zinc in reducing diarrhea duration and severity and maintaining intestinal mucosal integrity.

Poor intestinal repair is regarded as a key component of abnormal mucosal morphology. However, the exact factors underlying ineffective repair processes and continuing injury are understood poorly. The end result of mucosal derangement is poor absorption of luminal nutrients and increased permeability of the bowel to dietary or microbial antigens. Although PD is recognized widely as a nutritional disorder, there is remarkably poor understanding of the mechanisms underlying PD and the mucosal immunopathology in children who develop this syndrome. However, several factors that contribute to diarrheal persistence have been recognized, including general undernutrition, and micronutrient and immune deficiencies, suggesting that delayed intestinal repair following initial injury may be an important contributory factor. Figure 2 indicates the mechanisms associated with delayed intestinal repair and prolonged enteropathy that may underlie post-infectious PD.

A clear understanding of the alterations in intestinal morphology and physiology is crucial to the development of interventional strategies. However, a wide variety of post-PD pathological changes have been described by fairly small studies [33–35]. These studies indicate important findings suggestive of chronic inflammation and impaired mucosal integrity. In this regard there needs to be much more concerted work on representative populations.

Management of PD

The most important aspect in the management of the child with PD is an immediate assessment and triage for subsequent therapy. The management of PD in undernourished children is based on the principles of management of diarrhea and undernutrition. Although a subgroup may be severely undernourished requiring rapid nutritional rehabilitation, often in hospital, in other cases ambulatory management may be possible. Given the long time it may take to recovery, prolonged hospitalization may be quite problematic in developing countries, and whenever possible ambulatory or home-based therapy must be stressed.

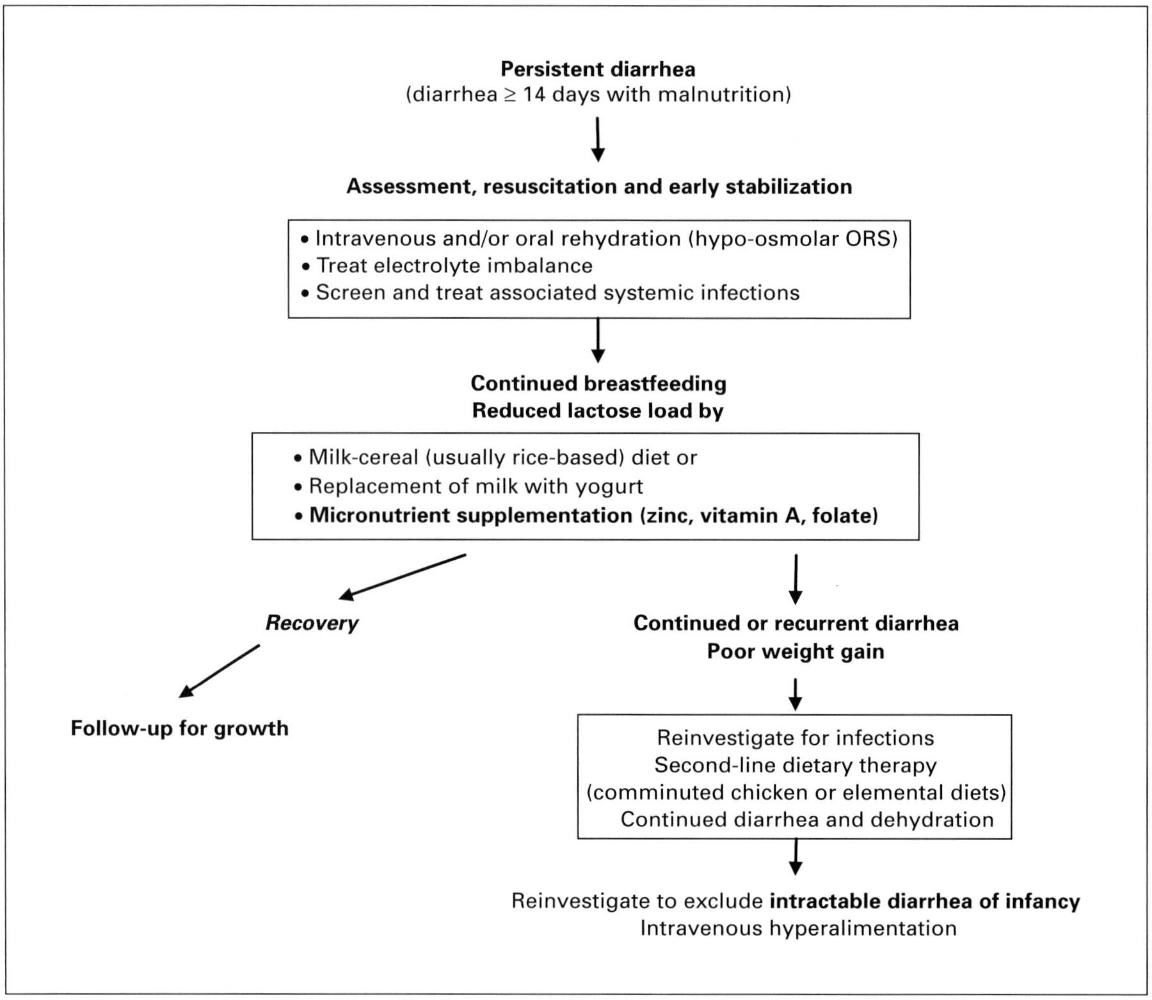

Fig. 3. Suggested algorithm for the management of persistant diarrhea.

The following represent the basic principles of management of PD and a suggested therapeutic approach is summarized in figure 3 [36].

(1) Initial Resuscitation and Stabilization

Most children with PD and associated undernutrition are not severely dehydrated and oral rehydration may be adequate. However, acute exacerbations and associated vomiting may require brief periods of intravenous rehydration with Ringer's lactate. Acute electrolyte imbalances such as hypokalemia and severe acidosis may require correction. More importantly, bacterial translocation [37] and systemic infections have been recognized in severely undernourished children with PD and are a frequent cause of early mortality. These must be screened for on admission. Up to half of all undernourished children with PD may have an associated systemic infection requiring resuscitation and antimicrobial therapy [38, 39]. In severely ill undernourished children requiring hospitalization, broad-spectrum antibiotics on initial admission and stabilization may be required while awaiting cultures. Some may also require empirical therapy for cryptosporidiosis, especially in HIV-infected children [40].

(2) Oral Rehydration Therapy

Although in general the standard WHO oral rehydration solution is adequate for replacing on-going losses, recent evidence indicates that low osmolality oral rehydration fluids [41, 42] may be advantageous in undernourished children, with no associated risk of hyponatremia.

(3) Enteral Feeding and Diet Selection

It is exceedingly rare to find PD in exclusively breastfed infants and, with the context specific possible exceptions of situations where PD accompanies perinatally acquired HIV infection, breastfeeding must be continued.

Despite mucosal abnormalities and diminution in digestive and absorptive mechanisms, most children with PD have adequate absorption capacity and tolerate enteral feedings. Metabolic balance studies in undernourished children with PD indicate that satisfactory carbohydrate, protein and fat absorption can take place on a variety of diets [43, 44]. In general, therefore, withdrawal of milk and replacement with specialized (and expensive) lactose-free formulations is unnecessary.

Most children with PD are not lactose intolerant, although administration of lactose loads exceeding 5 g/kg/day are associated with higher purging rates and treatment failures [45]. Alternative strategies of reducing lactose loads in undernourished children with PD include addition of milk to cereals and replacement of milk with fermented milk products such as yogurt. These dietary interventions have been evaluated extensively in several studies, and found to be efficacious and acceptable in comparison to several expensive formulations [7, 46].

Rarely when dietary intolerance precludes the administration of cow's milk-based formulations or cow's milk, it may be necessary to administer specialized milk-free diets such as a comminuted or blenderized chicken-based diet or an elemental formulation [47]. It must be pointed out that although effective in some settings [48], the latter are unaffordable in most developing countries. However, a guar gum-comminuted chicken combination has been found to be effective in children with PD [49]. In addition to the above, the addition of green banana or pectin to the diet [50] has been shown to be effective in the treatment of PD.

The usual energy density of any diet used for the therapy of PD should be around 1 kcal/g, aiming to provide an energy intake of at least 100 kcal/kg/day, and a protein intake of between 2 and 3 g/kg/day. The commonly used rice-lentil formulations in South Asia such as *khitchri* provide this energy density in combination with an optimal protein intake and amino acid ratio.

(4) Micronutrient Supplementation

It is recognized widely that most undernourished children with PD have associated deficiencies of micronutrients including zinc, iron and vitamin A. This may be a consequence of poor intake and continued enteral losses and requires replenishment during therapy [51]. Although the evidence supporting zinc administration in children with PD is persuasive, it is likely that these children have multiple micronutrient deficiencies. Concomitant vitamin A administration to children with PD was shown to improve outcomes [52, 53], especially in HIV endemic areas [54]. It is therefore important to ensure that all children with PD and undernutrition receive an initial dose of 100,000 units vitamin A and a daily intake of at least 3–5 mg/kg/day of elemental zinc.

(5) Follow-Up and Nutritional Rehabilitation in Community Settings

Given the high rates of relapse in most children with PD, it is important to address the underlying risk factors and institute preventive measures. These include appropriate feeding (breastfeeding and complementary feeding) and close attention to environmental hygiene and sanitation. This poses a considerable challenge in communities deprived of basic necessities such as clean water and sewage disposal.

In addition to preventive aspects, the challenge in most settings is to develop and sustain a form of dietary therapy using inexpensive, home-available and culturally acceptable ingredients that can be used to manage children with PD. Given that the majority of cases of PD occur in the community and that parents frequently are hesitant to seek institutional help, there is a need to develop and implement inexpensive and practical home-based therapeutic measures. Available evidence indicates that it may be entirely feasible to do so in community settings [55, 56].

Preventive Strategies for PD

Although optimal nutritional rehabilitation of children with PD is regarded as a cornerstone of management [44], prevention is critical. For this purpose large-scale improvements in diarrhea prevention and management strategies in developing countries are critical. As indicated by us in reviewing available child survival interventions, existing interventions can prevent almost 55% of all deaths globally in children under 5 years [57], a fifth of which are related to diarrhea.

These interventions include exclusive breastfeeding and safe complementary feeding strategies to prevent diarrhea and, in the event episodes occur, optimal management with improved oral rehydration, zinc supplementation and continued feeding. As indicated above, this requires that all episodes of diarrhea are recognized promptly and managed optimally with oral rehydration and enteral feeding with inexpensive, home-available and culturally acceptable diets that can be used to manage children with PD in ambulatory settings. The next steps would be to integrate these interventions so that families and community health workers can implement them in a variety of situations [58].

Providing essential preventive and therapeutic interventions to reduce PD in health systems are necessary in order to achieve the millennium development goals of reducing child mortality by two thirds by the year 2015. Early and unhygienic introduction of milks other than breast milk and recurrent acute diarrheal episodes that are managed poorly are important predisposing factors to the development of PD. It is important that these be prevented. These risk factors are generally prevalent in poor communities and both poverty alleviation and social sector support mechanisms are fundamentally important. Thus promotion of exclusive breastfeeding for at least 6 months, avoidance of unhygienic formula feeding, timely and adequate weaning with hygienic nutritious foods will help to prevent episodes of post-infectious PD. These must be coupled with environmental control measures and provision of safe water and safe foods [59]. In the absence of the latter, interventions to promote handwashing strategies and domestic measures to purify water are key to reducing the burden of diarrhea [60, 61].

A combination of allocation of appropriate resources for public health and basic needs, staff training and community mobilization are necessary to reduce the global burden of diarrhea and PD. This requires sustained and concerted efforts. In many parts of the developing world these interventions require that, apart from biomedical interventions, we give paramount importance to poverty alleviation and promotion of a human rights and equity agenda.

References

1 Black RE, Morris SS, Bryce J: Where and why are 10 million children dying every year? Lancet 2003;361:2226–2234.
2 Snyder JD, Merson MH: The magnitude of the global problem of acute diarrheal disease: a review of active surveillance data. Bull World Heath Organ 1982;60:605–613.
3 Bern C, Martines J, de Zoysa I, Glass RI: The magnitude of the global problem of diarrhoeal disease: a ten-year update. Bull World Health Organ 1992;70:705–714.
4 Yusufzai M, Bhutta ZA: Global burden of childhood diarrhea; in Bhutta ZA (ed): Contemporary Issues in Childhood Diarrhea and Malnutrition. Karachi, Oxford University Press, 2000, pp 1–22.
5 Kosek M, Bern C, Guerrant RL: The global burden of diarrheal disease as estimated from studies published between 1990 and 2000. Bull World Health Organ 2003;81:197–2004.
6 Anonymous: Persistent diarrhoea in children in developing countries: memorandum from a WHO Meeting. Bull World Health Organ 1988;66:709–717.
7 Anonymous: Evaluation of an algorithm for the treatment of persistent diarrhoea: a multicentre study. International Working Group on Persistent Diarrhoea. Bull World Health Organ 1996;74:479–489.
8 Schorling JB, Wanke CA, Schorlling SK, McAullife JF, de Souza MA, Guerrat RL: A prospective study of persistent diarrhea among children in an urban Brazilian slum: patterns of occurrence and etiologic agents. Am J Epidemiol 1990;132:144–156.
9 Fauveau V, Henry FJ, Briend A, Yunus M, Chakraborty J: Persistent diarrhea as a cause of childhood mortality in rural Bangladesh. Acta Paediatr Suppl 1992;381:12–14.
10 Victora CG, Huttly SRA, Fuch SC, et al: International differences in clinical patterns of diarrhoeal deaths: a comparison of children from Brazil, Senegal, Bangladesh and India. J Diarrhoeal Dis Res 1993;11:25–29.
11 Bhan MK, Bhandari N, Sazawal S, Clemens J, Raj P: Descriptive epidemiology of persistent diarrhoea among young children in rural northern India. Bull World Health Organ 1989;67:281–288.
12 Black RE: Persistent diarrhea in children of developing countries. Pediatr Infect Dis J 1993; 12:751–761.
13 Lima AAM, Fang G, Schorling JB, Albuquerque L, Mc Aulliffe JA, Mota S, Leite R, Guerrant RL: Persistent diarrhea in northeast Brazil: etiologies and interaction with malnutrition. Acta Paediatr Suppl 1992;381:39–44.
14 Moy RJ, Booth IW, Choto R-G, McNeish AS: Recurrent and persistent diarrhoea in a rural Zimbabwean community: a prospective study. J Trop Pediatr 1991;37:293–299.
15 Bhutta ZA, Ghishan F, Lindley K, Memon IA, Mittal S, Rhoads JM: Persistent and chronic diarrhea and malabsorption: Working Group report of the second World Congress of Pediatric Gastroenterology, Hepatology, and Nutrition. J Pediatr Gastroenterol Nutr 2004;(suppl 2):S711–S716.
16 Adejuyigbe EA, Oyelami O, Onayemi O, Durosinmi MA: Paediatric HIV/AIDS in Ile-Ife, Nigeria. Cent Afr J Med 2003;49:74–78.
17 Black RE, Brown KH, Becker S, Yunus M: Longitudinal studies of infectious diseases and physical growth of children in rural Bangladesh. I. Patterns of morbidity. Am J Epidemiol 1982;115:305–314.
18 Lanata CF, Black RE, Gilman RH, Lazo F, Del Aguila R: Epidemiologic, clinical, and laboratory characteristics of acute vs persistent diarrhea in periurban Lima, Peru. J Pediatr Gastroenterol Nutr 1991;12:82–88.
19 Mahmud A, Jalil F, Karlberg J, Lindblad BS: Early child health in Lahore, Pakistan: VII. Diarrhoea. Acta Paediatr Suppl 1993;390:79–85.
20 Haque R, Monda Dl, Kirkpatrick BD, Akther Farr BM, Sack RB, Petri WB Jr: Epidemiologic and clinical characteristics of acute diarrhea with emphasis on *Entamoeba histolytica* infections in preschool children in an urban slum of Dhaka, Bangladesh. Am J Trop Med Hyg 2003;69:398–405.
21 Ahmed F, Ansaruzzaman M, Haque E, Rao MR, Clemens JD: Epidemiology of postshigellosis persistent diarrhea in young children. Pediatr Infect Dis J 2001;20:525–530.
22 Hoglund P, Haila S, Socha J, Tomaszewski L, Saarialho-Kere U, Karjalainen-Lindsberg ML, Airola K, Holmberg C, de la CA, Kere J: Mutations of the Down-regulated in adenoma (DRA) gene cause congenital chloride diarrhoea. Nat Genet 1996;14:316–319.
23 Turk E, Zabel B, Mundlos S, Dyer J, Wright EM: Glucose/galactose malabsorption caused by a defect in the Na+/glucose cotransporter. Nature 1991;350:354–356.

24 Martin MG, Turk E, Lostao MP, Kerner C, Wright EM: Defects in Na+/glucose cotransporter (SGLT1) trafficking and function cause glucose-galactose malabsorption. Nat Genet 1996;12:216–220.
25 Naim HY, Roth J, Sterchi EE, Lentze M, Milla P, Schmitz J, Hauri HP: Sucrase-isomaltase deficiency in humans. Different mutations disrupt intracellular transport, processing, and function of an intestinal brush border enzyme. J Clin Invest 1988;82:667–679.
26 Amadi B, Kelly P, Mwiya M, Mulwazi E, Sianongo S, Changwe F, Thomson M, Hachungula J, Watuka A, Walker-Smith J, Chintu C: Intestinal and systemic infection, HIV, and mortality in Zambian children with persistent diarrhea and malnutrition. J Pediatr Gastroenterol Nutr 2001;32:550–554.
27 Baqui A H, Black R E, Sack R B, Chowdhury HR, Yunus M, Siddique A K: Malnutrition, cell-mediated immune deficiency and diarrhea: a community-based longitudinal study in rural Bangladeshi children. Am J Epidemiol 1993;137:355–365.
28 Azim T, Ahmad SM, Sefat-E-Khuda, Sarker MS, Unicomb LE, De S, Hamadani JD, Salam MA, Wahed MA, Albert MJ: Immune response of children who develop persistent diarrhea following rotavirus infection. Clin Diagn Lab Immunol 1999;6:690–695.
29 Taniguchi K, Rikimaru T, Yartey JE, Akpedonu P, Armar-Klemesu MA, Nkrumah FK, Kamiya H, Kishi K, Armar DA: Immunological background in children with persistent diarrhea in Ghana. Pediatr Int 1999;4:162–167.
30 Sazawal S, Black R E, Bhan M K, Bhandari N, Sinha A, Jalla S: Zinc supplementation in young children with acute diarrhea in India. N Engl J Med 1995;333:839–844.
31 Bhutta ZA, Bird SM, Black RE, Brown KH, Gardner JM, Hidayat A, Khatun F, Martorell R, Ninh NX, Penny ME, Rosado JL, Roy SK, Ruel M, Sazawal S, Shankar A: Therapeutic effects of oral zinc in acute and persistent diarrhea in children in developing countries: pooled analysis of randomized controlled trials. Am J Clin Nutr 2000;72:1516–1522.
32 WHO/UNICEF Joint Statement: Clinical Management of Acute Diarrhea. May 2004. http://www.mostproject.org/ZINC/WHO-UNICEF/Statement.pdf (accessed Feb 27, 2005).
33 Sullivan PB: Studies of the small intestine in persistent diarrhea and malnutrition: the Gambian experience. J Pediatr Gastroenterol Nutr 2002;34(suppl 1):S11–S13.
34 Campbell DI, Murch SH, Elia M, Sullivan PB, Sanyang MS, Jobarteh B, Lunn PG: Chronic T cell-mediated enteropathy in rural west African children: relationship with nutritional status and small bowel function. Pediatr Res 2003;54:306–311.
35 Fagundes-Neto U, De Martini-Costa S, Pedroso MZ, Scaletsky IC: Studies of the small bowel surface by scanning electron microscopy in infants with persistent diarrhea. Braz J Med Biol Res 2000;33:1437–1442.
36 Bhutta ZA: Persistent diarrhea; in Guandalini S (ed): Text Book of Gastroenterology. London, Taylor & Francis, 2004.
37 Campbell DI, Elia M, Lunn PG: Growth faltering in rural Gambian infants is associated with impaired small intestinal barrier function, leading to endotoxemia and systemic inflammation. J Nutr 2003;133:1332–1338.
38 Bhutta ZA, Nizami SQ, Thobani S: Factors determining recovery during nutritional therapy of persistent diarrhoea: the impact of diarrhoea severity and intercurrent infections. Acta Paediatr 1997;86:796–802.
39 Alam NH, Faruque AS, Dewan N, Sarker SA, Fuchs GJ: Characteristics of children hospitalized with severe dehydration and persistent diarrhoea in Bangladesh. J Health Popul Nutr 2001;19:18–24.
40 Amadi B, Mwiya M, Musuku J, Watuka A, Sianongo S, Ayoub A, Kelly P: Effect of nitazoxanide on morbidity and mortality in Zambian children with cryptosporidiosis: a randomised controlled trial. Lancet 2002;360: 1375–1380.
41 Sarker SA, Mahalanabis D, Alam NH, Sharmin S, Khan AM, Fuchs GJ: Reduced osmolarity oral rehydration solution for persistent diarrhea in infants: a randomized controlled clinical trial. J Pediatr 2001;138:532–538.
42 Dutta P, Mitra U, Dutta S, Manna B, Chatterjee MK, De A, Bhattacharya SK: Hypo-osmolar oral rehydration salts solution in dehydrating persistent diarrhoea in children: double-blind, randomized, controlled clinical trial. Acta Paediatr 2000;89:411–416.
43 Bhutta ZA, Molla AM, Isani Z, Badruddin S, Hendricks K, Snyder JD: Dietary management of persistent diarrhea: comparison of a traditional rice-lentil based diet with soy formula. Pediatrics 1991;88:1010–1018.
44 Bhutta ZA, Hendricks KH: Nutritional management of persistent diarrhea in childhood: a perspective from the developing world. J Pediatr Gastroenterol Nutr 1996;22:17–37.
45 Penny ME, Paredes P, Brown KH: Clinical and nutritional consequences of lactose feeding during persistent postenteritis diarrhea. Pediatrics 1989;84:835–844
46 Ashraf H, Ahmed S, Fuchs GJ, Mahalanabis D: Persistent diarrhoea: associated infection and response to a low lactose diet. J Trop Pediatr 2002;48:142–148.
47 Godard C, Bustos M, Munoz M, Nussle D: Value of a chicken-based formula for refeeding of children with protracted diarrhea and malnutrition in a developing country. J Pediatr Gastroenterol Nutr 1989;9:473–480.
48 Amadi B: Role of food antigen elimination in treating children with persistent diarrhea and malnutrition in Zambia. J Pediatr Gastroenterol Nutr 2002;34(suppl 1):S54–S56.
49 Alam NH, Meier R, Sarker SA, Bardhan PK, Schneider H, Gyr N: Partially hydrolysed guar gum supplemented comminuted chicken diet in persistent diarrhoea: a randomised controlled trial. Arch Dis Child 2005;90:195–199.
50 Rabbani GH, Teka T, Zaman B, Majid N, Khatun M, Fuchs GJ: Clinical studies in persistent diarrhea: dietary management with green banana or pectin in Bangladeshi children. Gastroenterology 2001;121:554–560.
51 Mahalanabis D, Bhan MK: Micronutrients as adjunct therapy of acute illness in children: impact on the episode outcome and policy implications of current findings. Br J Nutr 2001; 85(suppl 2):S151–S158.
52 Rahman MM, Vermund SH, Wahed MA, Fuchs GJ, Baqui AH, Alvarez JO: Simultaneous zinc and vitamin A supplementation in Bangladeshi children: randomised double blind controlled trial. BMJ 2001;323:314–318.
53 Khatun UH, Malek MA, Black RE, Sarkar NR, Wahed MA, Fuchs G, Roy SK: A randomized controlled clinical trial of zinc, vitamin A or both in undernourished children with persistent diarrhea in Bangladesh. Acta Paediatr 2001;90:376–380.
54 Villamor E, Mbise R, Spiegelman D, Hertzmark E, Fataki M, Peterson KE, Ndossi G, Fawzi WW: Vitamin A supplements ameliorate the adverse effect of HIV-1, malaria, and diarrheal infections on child growth. Pediatrics 2002;109:E6.
55 Bhandari N, Bahl R, Saxena M, Taneja S, Bhan MK: Prognostic factors for persistent diarrhoea managed in a community setting. Indian J Pediatr 2000;67:739–745.
56 Valentiner-Branth P, Steinsland H, Santos G, Perch M, Begtrup K, Bhan MK, Dias F, Aaby P, Sommerfelt H, Molbak K: Community-based controlled trial of dietary management of children with persistent diarrhea: sustained beneficial effect on ponderal and linear growth. Am J Clin Nutr 2001;73:968–974.
57 Jones G, R Steketee RW, Black RE, Bhutta ZA, Morris SS and the Bellagio Child Survival Study Group: How many child deaths can we prevent this year? Lancet 2003;362:65–71.
58 Travis P, Bennett S, Haines A, Pang T, Bhutta Z A, Hyder AA, Pielemeier NR, Mills A, Evans T: Overcoming health-systems constraints to achieve the Millennium Development Goals. Lancet 2004;364:900–906.
59 Sheth M, Obrah M: Diarrhea prevention through food safety education. Indian J Pediatr 2004;71:879–882.
60 Curtis V, Cairncross S: Effect of washing hands with soap on diarrhoea risk in the community: a systematic review. Lancet Infect Dis 2003;3: 275–281.
61 Luby SP, Agboatwalla M, Painter J, Altaf A, Billhimer WL, Hoekstra RM: Effect of intensive handwashing promotion on childhood diarrhea in high-risk communities in Pakistan: a randomized controlled trial. JAMA 2004;291: 2547–2554.